MASTER EDUCATOR

Exam Review

3rd Edition

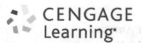
CENGAGE
Learning·

Australia • Brazil • Japan • Korea • Mexico • Singapore • Spain • United Kingdom • United States

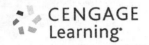

Exam Review for Master Educator
Milady

Vice President, Milady & Learning Solutions Strategy, Professional: Dawn Gerrain

Director of Content & Business Development, Milady: Sandra Bruce

Associate Acquisitions Editor: Philip I. Mandl

Product Manager: Maria Moffre-Barnes

Editorial Assistant: Elizabeth A. Edwards

Director, Marketing & Training: Gerard McAvey

Marketing Manager: Matthew McGuire

Senior Production Director: Wendy Troeger

Production Manager: Sherondra Thedford

Senior Content Project Manager: Nina Tucciarelli

Senior Art Director: Benj Gleeksman

For product information and technology assistance, contact us at **Cengage Learning Customer & Sales Support, 1-800-354-9706**

For permission to use material from this text or product, submit all requests online at **www.cengage.com/permissions**. Further permissions questions can be e-mailed to **permissionrequest@cengage.com**

Library of Congress Control Number: 2012956270

ISBN-13: 978-1-133-77659-8

ISBN-10: 1-133-77659-0

Milady
5 Maxwell Drive
Clifton Park, NY 12065-2919
USA

Cengage Learning is a leading provider of customized learning solutions with office locations around the globe, including Singapore, the United Kingdom, Australia, Mexico, Brazil, and Japan. Locate your local office at: **international.cengage.com/region**

Cengage Learning products are represented in Canada by Nelson Education, Ltd.

For your lifelong learning solutions, visit **milady.cengage.com**

Purchase any of our products at your local college store or at our preferred online store **www.cengagebrain.com**

Visit our corporate website at **cengage.com**.

Printed in the United States of America
8 9 10 11 12 13 14 22 21 20 19 18

Table of Contents

Part I
Basic Teaching Skills for Career Education Instructors

1 The Career Education Instructor

MULTIPLE CHOICE

1. Today's master educator will have qualities that will:
   a. facilitate learning.
   b. exhibit loyalty and fairness.
   c. demonstrate competency.
   d. all of the above. ____

2. To ensure a constructive working environment, your actions and performance will be:
   a. positive toward your employer and institution.
   b. negative toward the staff.
   c. sarcastic and demeaning of the institution.
   d. speaking ill of the students. ____

3. Upon receiving a license to teach, master educators will continue to gain new knowledge by:
   a. earning 20 continuing education credits.
   b. earning the minimum continuing education credits.
   c. earning 40 or more continuing education credits.
   d. earning 10 continuing education credits. ____

4. For educators to achieve recognition as authority figures, they must first have self-esteem and self-confidence. To hold someone in high esteem is to:
   a. be fashionably groomed.
   b. have no fear of failure.
   c. be honest with students.
   d. hold in high regard and prize accordingly. ____

5. The belief in one's own powers and abilities is called:
   a. skill development.   c. self-esteem.
   b. self-confidence.   d. ego. ____

6. Combined actions or an operation performed by a team, described by saying 1 + 1 = 3, is termed:
   a. synergy.   c. collaboration.
   b. teamwork.   d. fusion. ____

7. Being friends with students in a personal relationship outside the classroom may:
   a. disrupt the order that you have in your classroom.
   b. cause questions of fairness and equity.
   c. challenge your authority.
   d. all of the above. ____

8. Master educators will be aware of ethical standards and will:
   a. avoid criticism of others.
   b. keep confidentiality.
   c. instruct without prejudice and avoid unethical practices.
   d. all of the above. ____

9. Learning occurs when the classroom is:
   a. teacher centered.
   b. serious and student centered.
   c. teacher driven.
   d. student centered and fun. ____

10. The requirement for an educator to influence the classroom is:
    a. being a subject-matter expert.
    b. self-confidence and a climate for serious learning.
    c. high moral value.
    d. self-confidence and self-esteem. ____

11. Employers value educators who:
    a. wear the latest trend.
    b. have legible handwriting.
    c. require less supervision and have initiative.
    d. have good housekeeping skills. ____

12. Being prepared and planning lessons properly will assist the master educator in maintaining:
    a. correct pronunciation.   c. proper breathing.
    b. good posture.   d. self-control. ____

13. The responsibility of portraying a professional image rests with:
    a. the client.   c. sales clerks.
    b. the guest speaker.   d. educators.

14. To be just or fair so that the successive results or events are the same is called:
    a. consistency.   c. courtesy.
    b. compassion.   d. motivation. ____

15. The humane quality of understanding the suffering of others and wanting to do something about it is termed:
    a. courtesy.
    b. desire.
    c. consistency.
    d. compassion. ____

16. Good manners and polite behavior is termed:
    a. courtesy.
    b. consistency.
    c. compassion.
    d. desire. ____

17. External motivators will have little effect unless students are ready to:
    a. rebuke them.
    b. accept them.
    c. denounce them.
    d. refuse them. ____

18. To want something with a deep longing that impels people to believe that they can attain their goal is called:
    a. spiritualism.
    b. hard work.
    c. imagination.
    d. desire. ____

19. In your free time:
    a. associate with positive people.
    b. do things you enjoy doing.
    c. eliminate "I can't" from your vocabulary.
    d. all of the above. ____

20. Being a successful master educator will depend on your degree of:
    a. compassion.
    b. self-control.
    c. courtesy.
    d. self-motivation. ____

21. Which of the following is now believed by the medical profession to be a result of mental origin rather than physical in nature?
    a. bunions.
    b. carpal tunnel.
    c. fatigue.
    d. myopia. ____

22. Which of the following can help an educator become happier?
    a. exercise.
    b. maintaining a balanced diet.
    c. waking up singing.
    d. getting regular check-ups. ____

23. By introducing new ideas and activities daily, the master educator will ensure:
    a. returning students.
    b. late arrivals.
    c. high absenteeism.
    d. a large clinic. ____

24. Educators must be able to master communication with their students, who vary greatly in:
    a. age.
    b. background and attitude.
    c. culture and beliefs.
    d. all of the above. ____

25. Learners can provide you with a wealth of knowledge if you:
    a. speak your piece.
    b. put in your "two cents."
    c. let yourself be heard.
    d. keep an open mind. ____

26. An awkward moment may be turned into an insignificant moment if you:
    a. display poise and self-control.
    b. storm away.
    c. put the blame on someone else.
    d. cry. ____

27. Holding grudges can be:
    a. satisfying.
    b. harmful when applied to students.
    c. mind-boggling.
    d. proactive. ____

28. To develop a pleasant, enjoyable, gracious, and amiable personality:
    a. make the best of what you have.
    b. focus on the future rather than the past.
    c. don't live in fear.
    d. all of the above. ____

29. A group of peptide hormones that bind to opiate receptors and screen out unpleasant stimuli and reduce the experience of pain are called:
    a. tryptophans.
    b. serotonins.
    c. proteolytic enzymes.
    d. endorphins. ____

30. As a master educator you will radiate energy, good humor, and motivation because of:
    a. positive attitude.
    b. fashionable style.
    c. good character.
    d. perfect posture. ____

CHAPTER 2

The Teaching Plan and Learning Environment

MULTIPLE CHOICE

1. The twenty-first-century educator is better known as a(n):
   a. facilitator.
   b. educational consultant.
   c. teacher.
   d. instructor. ____

2. To better facilitate learning, the master educator will:
   a. use substandard equipment.
   b. gather materials as needed.
   c. identify the materials and equipment necessary for class.
   d. list necessary and unnecessary items. ____

3. Learning can be made easier if the classroom environment is:
   a. filled with aromatherapy.
   b. filled with an abundance of posters.
   c. organized and welcoming.
   d. both a and b. ____

4. The more time the educator spends in preparation, the more time the student has in:
   a. having services done.
   b. active learning.
   c. downtime.
   d. looking in trade journals. ____

5. An educator who has taken the time to organize and prepare the lesson will:
   a. develop handouts in a professional manner.
   b. review course material to refresh knowledge.
   c. organize needed materials, supplies, and educational aids.
   d. all of the above. ____

6. A data organization system ensures that:
   a. information will be available to you when needed.
   b. no one will find your materials.
   c. you have only electronic files.
   d. you have only hard-copy paper documents. ____

7. Students who feel that you have taken a personal interest in their success will:
   a. be absent.
   b. enjoy the educational experience.
   c. feel favoritism.
   d. study less.   ____

8. Confidentiality is a growing concern in our country. Which of the following protects privacy rights?
   a. Family Educational Rights and Parenting Act.
   b. Familial Endowment Rights and Privacy Agency.
   c. Federal Educational Rights and Privacy Act.
   d. Family Educational Rights and Privacy Act.   ____

9. School records should include a student's:
   a. learning objectives.   c. attitudes.
   b. attendance.   d. all of the above.   ____

10. A disorganized, cluttered, and poorly arranged classroom will cause:
    a. a negative impact on learning.
    b. stimulation and positive learning.
    c. positive reinforcement.
    d. higher-order thinking.   ____

11. Being able to put what you have learned into practical use, which is important to the goal-oriented adult learner, is called:
    a. imperative.   c. relevance.
    b. reverent.   d. immediate.   ____

12. Though adult learners may have established negative opinions about what is being taught, they are to:
    a. quietly follow the course of study.
    b. be actively involved in the learning process.
    c. do as they wish.
    d. be told their opinion doesn't matter.   ____

13. Master educators will keep lectures short, giving only essential information, because adult learners:
    a. sit passively.   c. need involvement.
    b. can use imagery.   d. learn through video only. ____

14. When you are creating a learning environment that facilitates various age groups working together, you are:
    a. giving a clinical experience.
    b. preparing a better workforce.
    c. practicing customer service.
    d. practicing state board skills. ____

15. Research tells us that there are differences between male and female students' participation in classroom discussion. Which of the following statements is true according to this research?
    a. Female students tend to keep speaking until they have no more to add to the conversation.
    b. Males have fewer words to say, but say them louder.
    c. Males tend to keep speaking when interrupted until their point is adequately made.
    d. Females are more demure in their speech. ____

16. Identity with or membership in a particular racial, national, or cultural group and observance of that group's customs, beliefs, and language is called:
    a. nationalism.   c. socialism.
    b. ethnicity.   d. none of the above. ____

17. To better acquaint yourself with your students' interests, past experiences, and attitudes and to get them involved in the learning process, you should:
    a. invite them to your office for interviews.
    b. talk to them individually while others wait.
    c. have them write a personal profile.
    d. both a and b. ____

18. The master educator will arrange the motivational classroom to allow for:
    a. more than one activity to occur.
    b. accessible materials and supplies.
    c. a clear view of all learners at all times.
    d. all of the above. ____

19. Color in an educational facility has an impact on the learner; for example, the color green gives us:
    a. a sense of security.   c. creativity.
    b. serenity.   d. both a and c. ____

20. Bulletin boards have many useful purposes, such as:
    a. being a mail box for students.
    b. enhancing student motivation.
    c. posting assignments and procedures.
    d. both b and c.   ____

21. Cultural differences may prove a challenge in the classroom;
    to avoid disparity the master educator will:
    a. honor ethnic differences.
    b. recognize cultural perspectives.
    c. stereotype students of different backgrounds.
    d. both a and b.   ____

22. Being familiar with the controls of the classroom's heating
    system, lighting, audio-visual equipment, and other
    equipment necessary for the smooth delivery of the lesson
    objectives is related to:
    a. the motivation technique.
    b. classroom maintenance.
    c. the physical environment.
    d. environmental protection.   ____

23. A seating arrangement suited for small classes and
    informal discussions that allows the facilitator to be seated,
    providing excellent use of eye contact, is the:
    a. semicircle arrangement.
    b. theater-style arrangement.
    c. classroom-style arrangement.
    d. boardroom style arrangement.   ____

24. The room arrangement that is conducive to lecture,
    demonstration, discussions, video projection, and group
    projects and also provides for a high degree of eye contact
    between the learners is the:
    a. amphitheater arrangement style.
    b. half-round or crescent style.
    c. circle arrangement style.
    d. U-shaped arrangement style.   ____

25. Students with documented disabilities are entitled to special accommodations under the:
    a. Accommodations for Americans with Disabilities Act of 1990.
    b. Diverse Learners of America Act of 1990.
    c. Americans with Disabilities Act of 1990.
    d. Americans for Diversity Act of 1990. ____

26. The main federal agency charged with the enforcement of safety and health legislation is the:
    a. Organization for Safety Administration.
    b. Occupational Safety and Health Administration.
    c. Oversight Committee for Safety and Health Agency.
    d. Occupational Health and Welfare Agency. ____

27. The school's hours of operation, required supervision, lab operations, rules for food and beverage consumption, check-out procedures, and supplies replacement information can be found in the school's:
    a. policies and procedures.   c. business cards.
    b. flyers.   d. entrance door. ____

28. In choosing a textbook you must consider whether:
    a. it meets the objectives of the course.
    b. it is too fundamental or too comprehensive.
    c. the reading level is appropriate.
    d. all of the above. ____

29. When selecting textbooks considerations should be made as to:
    a. timeliness.   c. author credibility.
    b. weight.   d. both a and c. ____

30. Two of the many responsibilities of a master educator are reporting to state agencies and record keeping for the institution; in order to be effective in these responsibilities the educator must be:
    a. serious.   c. thoughtful.
    b. confident.   d. accurate and current. ____

31. Attendance records must be accurately recorded for licensure and financial disbursement by which of the following agencies?
    a. State Board of Cosmetology.
    b. U.S. Department of Education.
    c. U.S. Financial Aid Department.
    d. Association of Beauty Schools. ____

32. One of the best ways to prevent student withdrawal from the program is:
    a. providing frequent downtime.
    b. having a sound orientation program.
    c. giving students time for services.
    d. having frequent guests. ____

33. Knowing who makes up the population of your class, their economic situations, and characteristics is called:
    a. demographics.   c. cultural.
    b. ethnicity.   d. humanity. ____

34. The use of color has been reported to have different effects on the brain. Blue has been identified as the color of:
    a. art.   c. academics.
    b. cuisine.   d. music. ____

35. Data conveyed in natural colors are retained by the brain at a much higher rate than those conveyed in:
    a. florescent colors.   c. black and white.
    b. pastel colors.   d. primary colors. ____

3 Teaching Study and Testing Skills

MULTIPLE CHOICE

1. It is possible to teach students:
   a. how to learn.
   b. that we are never too old to learn.
   c. that if we stop learning we stop growing.
   d. all of the above.   ____

2. A major barrier to learning is:
   a. the inability to read and study effectively.
   b. poor hygiene.
   c. ineffective listening.
   d. all of the above.   ____

3. A master educator will provide the necessary information for students to enhance their learning and will:
   a. develop handouts with tips on facilitating study.
   b. bring snacks to class.
   c. play music all the time in class.
   d. wear funny hats.   ____

4. When students are setting up a space for study it is important that the area:
   a. has proper temperature.
   b. has proper lighting.
   c. includes all necessary supplies and resources.
   d. all of the above.   ____

5. When students establish an organized study routine, they:
   a. are able to get to work on time.
   b. can service more clients.
   c. experience greater success.
   d. can leave early.   ____

6. Uninterrupted study time is important. Even students strong in musical/rhythmic intelligence should:
   a. turn off the MTV.
   b. take the phone off the hook.
   c. hang a DO NOT DISTURB sign.
   d. all of the above.   ____

7. When it comes to education the student must realize that:
   a. study time is a priority and comes first.
   b. study time is necessary but you need your fun first.
   c. fun is necessary to burn off all that energy; you can study afterward.
   d. once you have studied you won't have energy for fun. ____

8. Members of the educational team will be of benefit to you if they:
   a. discuss what is being learned and why.
   b. go about their day as usual.
   c. ask the learner questions that have no bearing on what they are learning.
   d. do nothing. ____

9. Be aware of the course you take with the learner; we should inspire, guide, motivate, and encourage and never:
   a. humor or nag.   c. pacify or overdo.
   b. nag or overdo.   d. appease or nag. ____

10. By providing positive reinforcement to students, the master educator is:
    a. giving them insincere praise.
    b. motivating the learners.
    c. building self-esteem.
    d. giving them sincere praise. ____

11. Helping students to recognize that everything in life is not always fair is:
    a. idealistic.   c. realistic.
    b. foolish.   d. impractical. ____

12. When reading difficult material, stress to the learner that:
    a. difficult material requires more time.
    b. playing soft music may help focus concentration.
    c. TV makes a good background.
    d. frequent breaks are necessary. ____

13. Before beginning to study, the student should survey the chapter by noting the:
    a. font.
    b. main ideas.
    c. length of the paragraphs.
    d. color of the font. ____

14. Relating what is being read to what has been previously learned in life and in school is referred to as:
   a. a memory.
   c. a camera eye.
   b. a flashback.
   d. a concept connector.   ____

15. Students using the highlighting pen have been using it with flourish; assist students to use color in note taking:
   a. with a system.
   b. with abandon.
   c. in 90 percent of the text.
   d. only at home.   ____

16. Students use a variety of note-taking methods to capture the major points of a lesson; as a master educator, remind students to:
   a. use Roman numerals.
   b. think about what they are hearing.
   c. use highlighting frequently.
   d. use paragraphs.   ____

17. Teaching study skills require the educator to assist the learner in developing ways to make learning easier, such as:
   a. designate and recognize cues.
   b. clarify information.
   c. use an organizational system.
   d. all of the above.   ____

18. For some learners the traditional method of outlining will not be an effective study skill; the master educator will employ the use of:
   a. mind mapping.
   c. fill-in-the-blank notes.
   b. paragraphing.
   d. word searches.   ____

19. When trying to retain information, students should select a time considered to be:
   a. the valley of enlightenment.
   b. peak performance time.
   c. the abyss of performance.
   d. the time to chill.   ____

20. To facilitate learning, students should:
   a. overeat for energy.
   b. stay up late to study.
   c. consider sleeping habits.
   d. push themselves even when tired.   ____

21. When motivation is low, the student should schedule:
    a. strenuous assignments.
    b. challenging tasks.
    c. complex material.
    d. less important study tasks.   ____

22. The master educator will encourage the student to consider
    the intricacy of an objective and devote:
    a. appropriate time to the task.
    b. time for socializing.
    c. time to influence teachers.
    d. attention to writing crib notes.   ____

23. When forming study habits, learners must be willing to:
    a. be responsible for their own learning.
    b. define their own personal values.
    c. logically prioritize goals.
    d. all of the above.   ____

24. We need consistency in our lives, and in our study habits as
    well. Show up for class, get assignments correct, and:
    a. rotate your place of study.
    b. establish a schedule.
    c. make excuses for missed assignments.
    d. arrive late for class.   ____

25. When you have a deviation from your schedule, it is best to:
    a. become agitated.
    b. become complacent.
    c. regroup and try again.
    d. grow fearful.   ____

26. What will aid your concentration as you set yourself to the
    goal of studying?
    a. adopting a mascot and developing a ritual.
    b. MTV.
    c. having a few friends over.
    d. getting involved in a new project.   ____

27. Many times when studying your mind may wander; the best
    thing to do is:
    a. plan a diversion.
    b. stand up and look away.
    c. leave the room.
    d. keep staring at the book.   ____

28. Master educators will promote a healthy alliance with the text and prevent book anxiety by:
    a. assisting students to associate the textbook with relaxation.
    b. teaching them that when they study, they should study, and when they worry they should worry; don't do both simultaneously.
    c. helping students find a comfortable spot where they can shift positions to help them relax.
    d. all of the above. ____

29. If we have done our job as master educators our students will relate the textbook with:
    a. fear.
    b. anxiety.
    c. relaxation.
    d. tension. ____

30. Barriers to success in learning include:
    a. skipping school.
    b. skipping homework.
    c. skipping mental presence.
    d. all of the above. ____

31. When a student chooses to avoid getting to know the educator or other students, this is known as:
    a. skipping mental presence.
    b. skipping relationships.
    c. skipping contention.
    d. skipping togetherness. ____

32. Master educators want learners to challenge fear; it is important to remember that:
    a. courage is the absence of fear.
    b. courage is being scared in the face of danger.
    c. courage is taking action in the face of fear.
    d. courage is facing pain. ____

33. A study group consists of like-minded students who gather to:
    a. share notes and prepare for class.
    b. review best-sellers.
    c. have an investment club.
    d. read the numismatic news. ____

34. When forming a study group:
    a. keep it to a minimum of four and a maximum of six.
    b. seek diversity but demand dedication.
    c. don't just invite friends.
    d. all of the above. ____

35. Every member of the study group is committed to the success of the group as a whole; therefore, in order to maintain integrity:
    a. eliminate members who are not serious.
    b. appoint a chairperson.
    c. establish guidelines.
    d. all of the above. ____

36. As a master educator you will have to communicate the importance of a balanced diet, sufficient pure water, and:
    a. shallow breathing.
    b. plenty of soda.
    c. staying free of drugs and alcohol.
    d. negative affirmations. ____

37. The factors that contribute to how well learners will perform on tests include:
    a. physical and psychological well-being.
    b. memory, note-taking skills, and test-taking skills.
    c. time management and reading skills.
    d. all of the above. ____

38. Test-taking skills are important because:
    a. if only some of the learners have test-taking skills and others do not, the test results may be invalid.
    b. test-wise learners may have less test anxiety.
    c. test-wise learners demand better results.
    d. all of the above. ____

39. In teaching effective test-taking skills, the master educator will ensure that all learners have an opportunity to:
    a. practice completing requested information.
    b. clearly understand the purpose of testing.
    c. be experienced in using testing materials.
    d. all of the above. ____

40. Preparation for the test does not begin the day before the test; learners must listen carefully in class and should also:

    a. begin to get mentally and physically ready.

    b. cram the night before.

    c. stay up late.

    d. eat junk food.   ____

41. On the day of the actual examination, if students have prepared in the manner that the master educator has suggested, they should:

    a. arrive early with the correct self-confident attitude; be alert, calm, and ready for the challenge.

    b. begin the test before reading all the directions and listening to the verbal instructions.

    c. take time to answer each question to their satisfaction, as they have ample time to take the test.

    d. be able to find skipped questions; there is no need to mark them and cause confusion.   ____

42. A strategy that allows learners to reach a logical conclusion by employing logical reasoning is referred to as:

    a. presumptive reasoning.

    b. obscure reasoning.

    c. deductive reasoning.

    d. hesitated reasoning.   ____

43. When studying the question stem, the learner should:

    a. look at the last word in the stem; the learner will know that the answer must begin with a vowel rather than a consonant.

    b. look for matches between the stem and one of the distracters or options.

    c. look at similar or related questions; they may provide clues.

    d. watch for qualifying conditions such as usually, commonly, never, and so forth.   ____

44. When giving advice to students about true/false testing, note that:

    a. they should consider wild exceptions to the statement.

    b. most statements are false.

    c. long statements are more likely to be false than short statements.

    d. for a statement to be true the entire statement must be true.   ____

45. Consider the following when teaching learners to answer multiple-choice items:
    a. do not select an answer that is grammatically incorrect.
    b. pay special attention to words such as *not, except,* and *but.*
    c. when two answers are close or similar, one is probably right.
    d. all of the above. ____

46. Strategies for essay questions include:
    a. brainstorm on paper before beginning to write your response.
    b. use flowery words to camouflage poor work.
    c. keep writing until the right answer comes to you.
    d. key words are just meant to overwhelm you. ____

47. Many times learners will prepare themselves for a test by following all the strategies that the master educator can provide, but will forget to:
    a. wear a watch, and get to the test site late.
    b. fill the gas tank of the car, or lock the keys inside.
    c. pace themselves, taking too much time on the first part of the test or on the more difficult questions.
    d. all of the above. ____

48. When master educators give a test, they will provide _____ for the learners
    a. instructions on marking the answer sheet correctly.
    b. candy for brain food.
    c. soft background music or rap.
    d. bottled water. ____

49. To reduce test anxiety, the master educator will be a positive and enthusiastic influence in the classroom and:
    a. control the noise level.
    b. keep the room cold to prevent illness.
    c. provide the answers.
    d. call a friend. ____

50. By developing effective study techniques, test-taking skills, and avoiding failure behaviors, learners and educators will:
    a. reduce the barriers to learning.
    b. achieve career success.
    c. reduce withdrawal rates at our nation's schools.
    d. all of the above. ____

4 Basic Learning Styles and Principles

MULTIPLE CHOICE

1. An individual's preferred method of thinking, understanding, and processing of information is called their:
   a. learning curve.
   b. learning style.
   c. intelligence quotient.
   d. preferred method of learning. ____

2. Diverse learners need more than sequential, analytical teaching; thus, the master educator will:
   a. vary teaching strategies.
   b. show more videos.
   c. play *Jeopardy*-type games.
   d. assign more projects. ____

3. Sensory learning styles include:
   a. seeing, hearing, and smelling.
   b. seeing, hearing, and talking.
   c. seeing, hearing, touching, and tasting.
   d. seeing, hearing, and touching. ____

4. The kinesthetic learner enjoys:
   a. reading alone.
   b. being physically involved.
   c. listening to lectures.
   d. nature. ____

5. Learning is a four-step process. The _____ step involves processing and understanding information.
   a. repetition   c. input
   b. desire   d. assimilation ____

6. The _____ step of the learning process involves practicing the underlying theory or practical application until the information or task has been mastered
   a. repetition   c. assimilation
   b. input   d. desire ____

7. When students receive information in an environment conducive to learning, it is called:
   a. assimilation.
   c. repetition.
   b. desire.
   d. input and environment. ____

8. What does Howard Gardner mean when he says that education is not unitary?
   a. Students can be smart in many ways.
   b. Students can be smart in only a few ways.
   c. Students learn in unison.
   d. Students can only learn in one way. ____

9. Howard Gardner has identified:
   a. six intelligences.
   c. eight intelligences.
   b. seven intelligences.
   d. nine intelligences. ____

10. The student who has the ability to successfully communicate, listen, read, write, and speak possesses:
    a. verbal/linguistic intelligence.
    b. body/kinesthetic intelligence.
    c. visual/spatial intelligence.
    d. musical/rhythmic intelligence. ____

11. When teaching the verbal linguistic learner:
    a. use metaphors, similes, and paraphrasing.
    b. assign journaling activities.
    c. employ word games, mnemonics, and affirmations.
    d. all of the above. ____

12. The ability to understand space and to comprehend and create images is related to the:
    a. verbal/linguistic intelligence.
    b. visual/spatial intelligence.
    c. body/kinesthetic intelligence.
    d. musical/rhythmic intelligence. ____

13. To appeal to visual/spatial learners, the master educator's lessons would include:
    a. lecture only.
    b. text readings.
    c. listening to tapes.
    d. designing graphic, logos, and flyers. ____

14. Color coding notes so that each topic is in the same color is extremely helpful for the:
    a. verbal/linguistic intelligence.
    b. logical/mathematical intelligence.
    c. visual/spatial intelligence.
    d. intrapersonal intelligence.   ____

15. Students who are good with sorting, classifying, sequencing, evaluating, and predicting display the:
    a. verbal/linguistic intelligence.
    b. visual/spatial intelligence.
    c. logical/mathematical intelligence.
    d. musical/rhythmic intelligence.   ____

16. When planning lessons with the logical/mathematical student in mind, include:
    a. evaluating ideas.
    b. classifying and categorizing information.
    c. making charts and graphs.
    d. all of the above.   ____

17. A logical/mathematical intelligence study tip would be to:
    a. study on the way to class.
    b. try not to reflect on the information.
    c. study in a cluttered area.
    d. study in a quiet place.   ____

18. Learners who would rather be left to their own resources, who think better on their own instead of bouncing ideas off others, possess:
    a. interpersonal intelligence.
    b. intrapersonal intelligence.
    c. environmental intelligence.
    d. naturalist intelligence.   ____

19. Activities that appeal to the intrapersonal intelligence include:
    a. working with small learning groups.
    b. assigning workbook activities.
    c. arranging Internet research projects.
    d. both b and c.   ____

20. During planning time, the master educator will use demonstrations or hands-on involvement to grasp the attention of the student with:
    a. bodily/kinesthetic intelligence.
    b. visual/spatial intelligence.
    c. logical/mathematical intelligence.
    d. verbal/linguistic intelligence. ____

21. To appeal to the bodily/kinesthetic intelligence:
    a. have students role-play.
    b. have students play charades.
    c. assign workbook activities.
    d. both a and b. ____

22. Study tips for the student with bodily/kinesthetic intelligence include:
    a. pace and recite while studying.
    b. use flashcards with another student.
    c. make notations of the chapter.
    d. both a and b. ____

23. The ability to relate to others, noticing their moods, motivations, and feelings, represents the:
    a. intrapersonal intelligence.
    b. naturalist intelligence.
    c. interpersonal intelligence.
    d. verbal/linguistic intelligence. ____

24. Activities to enhance the learning of students strong in the interpersonal intelligence include:
    a. team-building activities.
    b. working alone.
    c. individual workbook activities.
    d. journal writing. ____

25. The ability to comprehend and create meaningful sounds and the ability to keep rhythm is indicative of:
    a. verbal/linguistic intelligence.
    b. visual/spatial intelligence.
    c. bodily/kinesthetic intelligence.
    d. musical/rhythmic intelligence. ____

26. Having students write and perform musical jingles, put vocabulary into music or jingle format, and write a song including facts about the subject matter would be appropriate activities for students with strong:
    a. verbal/linguistic intelligence.
    b. musical/rhythmic intelligence.
    c. visual/spatial intelligence.
    d. naturalistic intelligence. ____

27. While studying, the musical/rhythmic intelligent student will be found:
    a. playing background music.
    b. beating out rhythms.
    c. writing a rap about the topic.
    d. all of the above. ____

28. Being able to make distinctions in the natural would and discriminate between natural and non-natural items is a trait of the:
    a. visual/spatial intelligence.
    b. verbal/linguistic intelligence.
    c. naturalist intelligence.
    d. bodily/kinesthetic intelligence. ____

29. The student with keen observational skills who can identify brands of cars, planes, sneakers, or handbags is strong in the:
    a. visual/spatial intelligence.
    b. naturalist intelligence.
    c. verbal/linguistic intelligence.
    d. bodily/kinesthetic intelligence. ____

30. Teaching activities that would interest the student with the naturalist intelligence include:
    a. listing natural ingredients in products.
    b. teaching aromatherapy.
    c. recording changes in hair, skin, or nails.
    d. all of the above. ____

31. When studying, the naturalist intelligent student might find satisfaction in:
    a. sorting and classifying subject matter.
    b. outdoor study when practical.
    c. taking a nature walk during study breaks.
    d. all of the above. ____

32. Knowing how we learn best enables students and educators to:
    a. make better choices.   **c.** study harder.
    b. use one intelligence.   **d.** read better. ____

33. Identifying all students' styles of learning will enable them to:
    a. look for a work environment that best suits them.
    b. receive better grades.
    c. none of the above.
    d. both a and b. ____

34. As master educators, we must present our teaching methodologies to:
    a. reach only intelligences like our own.
    b. reach all intelligences.
    c. reach ethnicities like ours.
    d. reach students with disabilities.

35. As long as the brain is still functioning, the age limit for developing in the interpersonal, intrapersonal, and logical/mathematical intelligences is:
    a. 50 to 60 years of age.   **c.** 70 to 80 years of age.
    b. 60 to 70 years of age.   **d.** no age limit. ____

36. When delivering lessons, the educator should attempt to reach at least:
    a. one or two intelligences in every class.
    b. two or three intelligences in every class.
    c. three or four intelligences in every class.
    d. four or five intelligences in every class. ____

37. During the course of the week, educators should have addressed:
    a. four or five of the intelligences.
    b. five or six of the intelligences.
    c. six or seven of the intelligences.
    d. all of the intelligences. ____

38. The standard IQ (intelligence quotient) test measures:
   a. verbal/linguistic and bodily/kinesthetic intelligences.
   b. verbal/linguistic and logical/mathematical intelligences.
   c. musical/rhythmic intelligence.
   d. interpersonal intelligence.   ____

39. Our students' learning styles may change due to:
   a. circumstances.   **c.** time of day.
   b. subject matter.   **d.** both a and b.   ____

40. As a master educator, you have the ability to enhance the brain power of your students by:
   a. delivering content that reaches all intelligences.
   b. giving IQ tests.
   c. keeping accurate test scores.
   d. maintaining student data.   ____

CHAPTER 5

Basic Methods of Teaching and Learning

MULTIPLE CHOICE

1. The art of imparting knowledge or instruction by precept, example, or experience is the realm of the:
   - **a.** lawyer.
   - **b.** teacher.
   - **c.** nurse.
   - **d.** nutritionist. _____

2. To increase learners' understanding of the material presented, they must:
   - **a.** take action on the material.
   - **b.** see the material.
   - **c.** hear the material.
   - **d.** listen to music while the material is presented. _____

3. The essential steps in learning are:
   - **a.** desire, information, assimilation, and repetition.
   - **b.** desire, information, intelligence, and repetition.
   - **c.** desire, information, assimilation, and interest.
   - **d.** desire, affirmation, assimilation, and repetition. _____

4. The manner in which educators use the materials and resources available to them to produce or achieve the desired objectives and facilitate learning for all students is termed as:
   - **a.** presentation.
   - **b.** teaching method.
   - **c.** learning objective.
   - **d.** teaching standard. _____

5. In order for the learner to receive the information, the teaching methods must be:
   - **a.** appropriate for the lesson.
   - **b.** appropriate for the type and age of the learner.
   - **c.** varied within the class.
   - **d.** all of the above. _____

6. A discourse or formal presentation conveying information, explaining facts, or describing procedures is called a(n):
   - **a.** demonstration.
   - **b.** lecture.
   - **c.** illustrated talk.
   - **d.** none of the above. _____

7. When delivering a lesson in the lecture mode:
   a. be brief.
   b. keep it lengthy.
   c. the duration is of no consequence.
   d. all of the above. ____

8. The demonstration method is used to:
   a. break the monotony of the classroom.
   b. show off the educator's skills.
   c. illustrate correct procedures.
   d. none of the above. ____

9. When giving an interactive lecture the master educator will:
   a. incorporate a closing for the presentation that has a high impact on the learners.
   b. stand in the front of the class and look at the board while lecturing.
   c. direct the students to read aloud from their textbook.
   d. give the students time to answer workbook questions. ____

10. Identifying the objectives of the lesson, motivating the students, gathering materials and tools ahead of time, and ensuring that students have unobstructed views is part of the lesson:
   a. preparation.   c. questioning.
   b. opening.   d. closure. ____

11. During a demonstration, the master educator will perform the procedure:
   a. with full speed ahead to show students how it will be done in the clinic or work environment.
   b. extremely slowly.
   c. at an appropriate speed that ensures students do not miss key steps.
   d. along with a video presentation. ____

12. Master educators will react to nonverbal clues of disinterest by:
   a. stopping the lesson and calling attention to the students' inappropriateness.
   b. stopping the lesson and assigning workbook activities.
   c. varying the stimuli by changing the activity.
   d. starting a different lesson. ____

13. Passing objects during a demonstration will:
    a. enhance learning.
    b. allow the student to see the object up close.
    c. allow students to feel the object.
    d. detract the learners from important steps
       in the demonstration.   ____

14. Providing the opportunity for learners to practice the skill
    demonstration soon after its presentation is termed:
    a. clinic.   c. practice.
    b. application.   d. both b and c.   ____

15. To ensure that a learner's practice makes procedures
    permanent, the master educator will:
    a. give assistance.
    b. closely supervise student practice.
    c. give immediate feedback.
    d. all of the above.   ____

16. Group discussion and discovery is extremely advantageous
    because it:
    a. lacks immediate feedback.
    b. encourages social interaction.
    c. requires a high degree of learner participation.
    d. both b and c.   ____

17. To ensure the best results in group discussion and
    discovery:
    a. require that opinions and statements brought forth by
       the learners be supported by facts.
    b. allow for differences of opinions among learners.
    c. avoid interrupting learners and groups when at work.
    d. all of the above.   ____

18. Role-play is an effective way for learners to observe:
    a. other students at play.
    b. a comedy in the classroom.
    c. how various conflict situations should be handled.
    d. the educator dealing with conflict.   ____

19. During role-play, those observing should be:
   a. working in workbooks.
   b. analyzing the enactment and taking notes for discussion.
   c. studying for upcoming tests.
   d. watching the role-play only. ____

20. When using role-play as a teaching method:
   a. use learners' personal problems.
   b. it is not necessary to plan ahead.
   c. it is not necessary to have students volunteer.
   d. select situations that will not embarrass any of the learners. ____

21. The learner should leave the role-play experience feeling:
   a. that there is only one way to solve a conflict.
   b. that there is likely more than one solution to any conflict.
   c. discouraged about handling conflicts.
   d. that role-play is a waste of time. ____

22. The technique of hand-sketching visual images into the squares of a matrix is called:
   a. mind mapping.   **c.** window paning.
   b. sequencing blocks.   **d.** brick patterns. ____

23. Because research states that the memory can retain only certain bits of information, window paning contains:
   a. six panes.   **c.** eight panes.
   b. seven panes.   **d.** nine panes. ____

24. The master educator sees field trips as being important to the learners':
   a. self-discovery.   **c.** career path.
   b. active learning.   **d.** all of the above. ____

25. After the scheduled field trip and an organized review of the students' observations, the master educator will:
   a. tie those observations to the stated objectives identified for the field trip.
   b. listen attentively.
   c. take notes for distribution at a later time.
   d. commend students for being observant and cooperative. ____

26. Having a preliminary meeting with a guest speaker is recommended so that:
    a. you can meet and greet the speaker.
    b. you can write what you want the speaker to say.
    c. you can lay the ground rules for the presentation.
    d. none of the above. ____

27. While the guest speaker is presenting to the learners, it is the perfect opportunity for the master educator to:
    a. catch up on paperwork.
    b. take a short break.
    c. work on the supply room.
    d. none of the above. ____

28. It may be necessary for the master educator to assist the guest speaker in:
    a. getting learners involved.   c. presentation tips.
    b. taking control of the class.   d. all of the above. ____

29. Mind mapping is a significant method of learning for the:
    a. musical learner.   c. visual learner.
    b. verbal learner.   d. linguistic learner. ____

30. Mind mapping can be more effective than:
    a. using workbooks.   c. outlining chapters.
    b. using textbooks.   d. crossword puzzles. ____

31. Mind mapping:
    a. is difficult to learn.
    b. is complicated to learn and takes hours of time.
    c. needs the input of more than one student.
    d. is easy to learn and may be organized in a matter of minutes. ____

32. By depicting images or pictures throughout the mind map it:
    a. creates a cartoon for the learner.
    b. aids in recall.
    c. stimulates both sides of the brain.
    d. both b and c. ____

33. Individualized feedback can be received on a regular basis by using:
    a. testing.   c. student interaction.
    b. peer coaching.   d. computer software. ____

34. Projects have their place in the educational arena and they can be very effective in:
  a. filling the time.
  b. making the students look busy.
  c. the use of arts and crafts.
  d. developing problem-solving skills. _____

35. To be effective, workbook assignments should:
  a. be completely filled in.
  b. follow the lesson or text material being covered.
  c. not be used for all learner types.
  d. none of the above. _____

36. Case studies should be directly related to:
  a. conflicts in the class.   **c.** the male gender.
  b. the female gender.   **d.** objectives of the lesson. _____

37. When developing questions for the case studies, the most difficult question should be placed:
  a. first.   **c.** in the middle.
  b. second.   **d.** last. _____

38. There are two types of case studies; one presents only the problem and the other:
  a. presents the problem with one possible solution to the problem.
  b. presents the problem with two possible solutions to the problem.
  c. presents the problem with three possible solutions to the problem.
  d. presents the problem with four possible solutions to the problem. _____

39. Provide a link between the student's skill and the information being taught is a method termed:
  a. bridging.   **c.** dove-tailing.
  b. linking.   **d.** concept connectors. _____

40. Providing links with the learners' past experiences and the objective of the lesson being taught is called:
  a. bridging the gap.   **c.** linking.
  b. concept connectors.   **d.** chain linking. _____

41. The process whereby the mind forms a mental image of the one performing the objectives of the lesson is termed:
    a. imagination.
    c. visualization.
    b. dreaming.
    d. mind-wandering. ____

42. Students remain focused on the lesson when educators enhance the lesson with meaningful:
    a. periodical personal anecdotes.
    b. lectures.
    c. notes.
    d. handouts. ____

43. Songs, words, or phrase associations that will trigger the recall of key information are called:
    a. acronyms.
    c. alphabetisms.
    b. mnemonics.
    d. synonyms. ____

44. When there is a "sag" during a class of heavy content material, the master educator will use:
    a. energizers.
    b. workbook activities.
    c. fill-in-the-blank worksheets.
    d. none of the above. ____

45. Energizers are brief activities that take:
    a. one to three minutes.
    c. five to seven minutes.
    b. three to five minutes.
    d. seven to nine minutes. ____

46. Experimentation is a great way to reach:
    a. intuitive learners.
    c. introverted learners.
    b. shy learners.
    d. all of the above. ____

47. Master educators should incorporate humor into the presentations:
    a. constantly.
    c. only when planned.
    b. to make a point.
    d. both a and c. ____

48. Humor used in the classroom must:
    a. be sarcastic and bold.
    b. have nothing to do with the presentation.
    c. be relevant and fit naturally and logically into the presentation.
    d. have a punch line that incorporates politics. ____

49. To maximize participation of all group members, the master educator will limit groups to:

   a. five members.   **c.** seven members.

   b. six members.   **d.** eight members. ____

50. The master educator will only take over the group discussions when:

   a. there is a question.

   b. the material seems confusing.

   c. students are at a roadblock.

   d. none of the above. ____

6 Communicating Confidently

MULTIPLE CHOICE

1. Sharing your knowledge with the students is what becoming a master educator is all about; but, you remain an ineffective educator if you cannot:
   a. use a laptop computer.
   b. use a smartboard.
   c. recite the cranial nerves from memory.
   d. effectively communicate. ____

2. The transfer of information can occur in a variety of ways, through the spoken or written word or nonverbally through:
   a. body language.
   c. facial expressions.
   b. gestures.
   d. all of the above. ____

3. Information that we send without the use of words is referred to as:
   a. Morse code.
   c. body language.
   b. Braille.
   d. sign language. ____

4. When nonverbal communication is added to spoken or verbal communication:
   a. the meaning is enhanced or changed.
   b. the meaning stays the same.
   c. the verbal communication says more.
   d. the nonverbal communication makes no difference. ____

5. The way the master educator packages the words of a message to the learner is called:
   a. coding.
   c. decoding.
   b. encoding.
   d. receiving. ____

6. To complete the communication process, the receiver of the sender's information must be able to:
   a. code it.
   c. decode it.
   b. encode it.
   d. receive it. ____

7. Speaking does not necessarily mean we can communicate; master educators will find communication barriers that can be classified as:
   - **a.** physical.
   - **b.** mental and emotional.
   - **c.** cultural.
   - **d.** all of the above. ____

8. A disturbing factor in the environment that prevents full communication, such as room temperature, noise, or distracting activities, is called a(n):
   - **a.** physical barrier.
   - **b.** mental barrier.
   - **c.** emotional barrier.
   - **d.** cultural barrier. ____

9. An assumption made based on previous knowledge or experience by one party that the information would be dull would be referred to as a(n):
   - **a.** physical barrier.
   - **b.** mental barrier.
   - **c.** emotional barrier.
   - **d.** cultural barrier. ____

10. Traditions, manners, and habits may create distance in a speaker–listener relationship; this is a(n):
    - **a.** physical barrier.
    - **b.** mental barrier.
    - **c.** emotional barrier.
    - **d.** cultural barrier. ____

11. Stress, worry, fear, anger, and prejudices can restrict effective communication; this is called a(n):
    - **a.** physical barrier.
    - **b.** mental barrier.
    - **c.** emotional barrier.
    - **d.** cultural barrier. ____

12. Research shows that only 7 percent of the message we want to communicate is accomplished through the words we speak; how we say the words determines:
    - **a.** 18 percent.
    - **b.** 28 percent.
    - **c.** 38 percent.
    - **d.** 48 percent. ____

13. It is our appearance and posture, our facial expressions, our gestures, and our eye contact that comprise the remaining _____ of our communication tools.
    - **a.** 55 percent
    - **b.** 58 percent
    - **c.** 65 percent
    - **d.** 68 percent ____

14. The way we say things will tell the listener what mood we are experiencing at the time; this fluctuation in our voice is known as:
    - **a.** clarity.
    - **b.** intonation.
    - **c.** cadence.
    - **d.** consonance. ____

15. Master educators know that the clarity of speech will greatly influence the effectiveness of our communication; thus, we must make every effort to:
- **a.** articulate.
- **b.** emulate.
- **c.** have good pitch.
- **d.** be eloquent.

_____

16. Students will model the educators, especially when learning terms that are not familiar to them. Therefore, we must pronounce our words correctly; this is:
- **a.** intonation.
- **b.** cadence.
- **c.** enunciation.
- **d.** emphasis.

_____

17. We can determine people's state of mind from:
- **a.** their facial expression.
- **b.** the way they drive.
- **c.** their walk.
- **d.** the way they stand.

_____

18. When you see learners avoiding eye contact:
- **a.** they are playing shy.
- **b.** they don't want to be called on.
- **c.** they are going to surprise you with the right answer.
- **d.** all of the above.

_____

19. Master educators will remember cultural differences, such as the following:
- **a.** looking down to avoid eye contact is just a habit.
- **b.** some cultures find eye gazing disrespectful.
- **c.** looking downward is a sign of respect.
- **d.** all of the above.

_____

20. Teaching client consultation is one of the most important skills to facilitate. Students should learn that:
- **a.** it does not matter where you do the client consultation as long as you do it.
- **b.** the styling mirror works fine, because you can see the back of the client and also give makeup tips.
- **c.** they must use the mirror when doing client consultations.
- **d.** face-to-face consultations will work best rather than consultations through the styling mirror.

_____

21. Master educators can use gestures in the classroom:
- **a.** for clarity.
- **b.** for size or shape.
- **c.** for location.
- **d.** all of the above.

_____

22. When someone is standing too close we get uncomfortable; the correct comfort zone for social distance where the average person feels comfortable is:

a. 12 to 18 inches.
b. 18 to 24 inches.
c. 24 to 30 inches.
d. 30 to 36 inches. ____

23. We enter the intimate zone when we touch another person; this area extends:

a. 6 to 10 inches.
b. 10 to 14 inches.
c. 14 to 18 inches.
d. 18 to 24 inches. ____

24. The two groups of body language postures are known as:

a. forward/back and open/closed.
b. reflective/reposed.
c. combative/reposed.
d. reflective/composed. ____

25. A person who is accepting the messages being sent, with arms open and legs uncrossed, is exhibiting:

a. forward/back posture.
b. open/closed posture.
c. forward/open posture.
d. back/closed posture. ____

26. When the listener is leaning forward and pointing at the speaker, he or she is exhibiting:

a. forward/back posture.
b. open/closed posture.
c. open/back posture.
d. forward/closed posture. ____

27. The open/forward mode indicates the listener is actively engaged and it would be an appropriate time to "close the sale." This body language is:

a. combative.
b. fugitive.
c. reflective.
d. responsive. ____

28. People in the open/back mode are interested and receptive but not actively accepting the information; they are feeling:

a. combative.
b. fugitive.
c. reflective.
d. responsive. ____

29. The closed/back mode suggests that the listener is trying to escape; use tactics to spark interest because the learner is feeling:

a. combative.
b. fugitive.
c. reflective.
d. responsive. ____

30. If the listener is likely to present active resistance and is closed/ forward, you will need to defuse the anger and make every attempt to avoid a confrontation. This is definitely the:
    a. combative mode.
    c. reflective mode.
    b. fugitive mode.
    d. responsive mode. ____

31. To be an effective active listener and benefit the learner you will:
    a. interrupt the speaker for clarification.
    b. focus on what is being said, and if your mind drifts, just look like you are listening.
    c. reflect on what has been said and paraphrase it.
    d. all of the above. ____

32. The degree to which a person is open in his or her dealings with others is termed:
    a. consequential.
    c. assertiveness.
    b. amenable.
    d. responsiveness. ____

33. A mode of communication that shows a degree of boldness or confidence in dealing with others is referred to as:
    a. responsiveness.
    c. aggressiveness.
    b. assertiveness.
    d. proactiveness. ____

34. People who are guarded in their interaction with others, are not outgoing, tend to be reserved in revealing personal information, and value self-control are referred to as:
    a. achievers.
    c. sellers.
    b. relaters.
    d. thinkers. ____

35. These communicators score high in the self-control department and resist revealing too much information about the inner self; however, they are very assertive and express their expectations clearly.
    a. achievers.
    c. sellers.
    b. relaters.
    d. thinkers. ____

36. A person who often will tell you about accomplishments and ambitions and is warm and friendly is the communicator who is:
    a. the achiever.
    c. the seller.
    b. the relater.
    d. the thinker. ____

37. Communicators who are less concerned about themselves than the receivers and will ask personal questions are known as:
   a. achievers.
   c. sellers.
   b. relaters.
   d. thinkers. ____

38. Using what you know about communication styles will:
   a. identify potential communication problems.
   b. lead to action to improve rapport with listeners.
   c. improve the quality of your communication.
   d. all of the above. ____

39. A technique used to build rapport by being more alike in communication and imitating in some small, subtle instance another's behavior to create harmony is referred to as:
   a. copying.
   c. reflecting.
   b. mirroring.
   d. resembling. ____

40. The ways in which nonverbal communication can be mirrored include eye contact and:
   a. posture.
   c. gestures.
   b. facial expressions.
   d. all of the above. ____

41. When feeling self-conscious, a coping strategy is to:
   a. concentrate on your purpose.
   b. take the focus off yourself; occupy yourself with a task.
   c. take deliberate control of your thoughts.
   d. all of the above. ____

42. Learning to speak properly gives you a great deal of confidence; it also:
   a. causes others to respect you.
   b. makes communication clearer.
   c. gives you self-respect.
   d. all of the above. ____

43. To make classes more interesting a master educator will become an accomplished storyteller by developing:
   a. anecdotes.
   c. puns.
   b. jokes.
   d. one-liners. ____

44. Becoming a skilled communicator takes practice; confidence builders include:
   a. answer with a unique response.
   b. ask pleasing questions.
   c. talk less; listen more.
   d. all of the above. ____

45. When communicating with others, interjecting phrases like, "I agree" or "Yes, that's right" is a form of:
   a. appeasement.
   b. positive reinforcement.
   c. capitulation.
   d. surrender. ____

46. Even though the school community is usually close-knit, it is important for you to:
   a. be professional and get very tight knit with personnel.
   b. be professional and keep your distance.
   c. be professional and maintain boundaries.
   d. be professional and keep them guessing. ____

47. We cannot pick whom we work with; in all cases we must come to the workplace and:
   a. remain objective.
   b. treat everyone with respect.
   c. be honest and sensitive.
   d. all of the above. ____

48. The individual who has the responsibility for daily maintenance and operation of the school and student and client service is the:
   a. counselor.
   b. educator.
   c. manager.
   d. receptionist. ____

49. When bringing an issue to the manager, bring some possible solutions along to indicate that you:
   a. are working in the best interest of the school.
   b. are working toward a higher pay raise.
   c. are working at a possible change in job status.
   d. do not have much to do and had lots of time to do research. ___

50. Going to the manager with information that is not accurate is wasting time; when seeing the manager:
   a. get your facts straight.
   b. be open and honest.
   c. do not complain about colleagues.
   d. all of the above. ____

CHAPTER 7

Effective Presentations

MULTIPLE CHOICE

1. When you send and receive information you are:
   a. communicating.
   b. conversing.
   c. listening.
   d. all of the above.
   ____

2. Our classrooms have a variety of cultures, including some students for whom English is a second language. When delivering lessons:
   a. use slang; everyone understands it.
   b. speak as you normally would; quickly is fine.
   c. shout, as this helps remove the language barrier.
   d. speak clearly and concisely.
   ____

3. CREATE is an acronym that stands for:
   a. consider, research, examples, analyze, teach.
   b. create, research, edit, analog, teach.
   c. contemplate, reproach, examine, apply, teach.
   d. change, respect, examine, analyze, topics.
   ____

4. With consideration of the topic in mind, the educator will determine:
   a. how much time will be needed for the presentation.
   b. the physical environment in which the lesson will be presented.
   c. how much prior knowledge the students may already have about the topic.
   d. all of the above.
   ____

5. Since the master educator is considered a subject-matter expert in every category within a program, it would be appropriate to:
   a. deliver the lesson from memory.
   b. use lesson plans that have not been updated.
   c. research each topic.
   d. interject humor that may not address the lesson.
   ____

6. By citing examples for clarification, the master educator will bring clarity and meaning to the points delivered without:
   a. being misunderstood by anyone.
   b. making inappropriate remarks.
   c. conducting himself improperly.
   d. all of the above.
   ____

7. Watching the students as the educator prepares for the classroom presentation and making mental notes on their reactions and body language can be best described as:
   a. "Analyze Your Learners."   c. "Snap, Crackle, Pop."
   b. "Stop, Camera, Action."   d. "Analysis 101."   ____

8. Because master educators must present themselves before classes each day, it is important to:
   a. teach with poise.
   b. wear fashionable heels.
   c. wear trendy makeup.
   d. show up in the best car on the lot.   ____

9. When speaking, the master educator will give thought to:
   a. rate.   c. tone.
   b. pitch.   d. all of the above.   ____

10. To have credibility with the students, the master educator must convey:
    a. poise.   c. self-assurance.
    b. confidence.   d. all of the above.   ____

11. Educators who enter the classroom with enthusiasm will:
    a. meet with enthusiastic students.
    b. be exhausted at the end of the day.
    c. make students nervous.
    d. eventually lose their enthusiasm.   ____

12. Master educators who are thoroughly prepared prior to entering the classroom will:
    a. be tense and nervous.
    b. be relaxed and enjoy the students.
    c. have control issues.
    d. be insecure.   ____

13. To build a lasting impression on learners, master educators will:
    a. enter the classroom with firmness and resolve.
    b. be determined to get the objective across to their students in the manner of a drill sergeant.
    c. believe in what they are saying and be enthusiastic.
    d. none of the above.   ____

14. The mnemonic that assists the master educator in preparing a dynamic lesson is:
   a. BUILD.
   c. SHAPE.
   b. FRAME.
   d. CREATE. ____

15. When the students are not ready to receive the message the educator is sending, the educator should:
   a. apply discipline.
   b. end the class.
   c. tune in to WII-FM (What's In It For Me?).
   d. assign busywork. ____

16. The need to feel a certain degree of control or mastery over others is the need for:
   a. financial security.
   b. pride and importance.
   c. approval and recognition.
   d. personal power. ____

17. People need to enjoy ego gratification and a feeling of importance; this is called the need for:
   a. approval and recognition.
   c. personal power.
   b. pride and importance.
   d. desire to win. ____

18. Our need for the opportunity to express our creativity and feel that we have contributed something worthwhile is the need for:
   a. accomplishment and creative expression.
   b. pride and importance.
   c. approval and recognition.
   d. self-esteem, love, and emotional security. ____

19. Our need to experience love in all forms, be emotionally secure, and respect ourselves is the need for:
   a. sense of belonging.
   b. pride and importance.
   c. approval and recognition.
   d. self-esteem, love, and emotional security. ____

20. When educators make themselves available to students early in the day, during breaks, and after class, they:
   a. should ask for more pay.
   b. waste valuable time.
   c. establish strong personal contact.
   d. should be home. ____

21. By being aware of the classroom environment and the students' comfort, varying the stimuli, using partially completed handouts, and encouraging questions in class master educators are:
    a. getting the learners in an active learning mood.
    b. making too much work for themselves.
    c. making the learners anxious and upset over all they must accomplish.
    d. making other educators in the school look bad. ____

22. Personal anecdotes interjected in the presentation will:
    a. build rapport with the learners.
    b. support the content.
    c. humanize the content.
    d. all of the above. ____

23. Avoid giving any criticism to any student:
    a. at any time.   c. in public.
    b. without a witness.   d. in an empty classroom. ____

24. Some students feel embarrassed about asking questions; thus, the master educator will address incorrect responses from students in a manner that does not humiliate the students and will:
    a. embarrass them.
    b. cause them to think before asking another question.
    c. encourage questions and feedback.
    d. all of the above. ____

25. Learning to measure where the learners are and where they would like to be is encouraging:
    a. personal competition.   c. anxiety attacks.
    b. frustration.   d. tension. ____

26. Identifying long-term benefits and stressing the value of internal motives will:
    a. assist learners in mastering information and skills being presented.
    b. discourage learners from searching for their own motivation.
    c. allow learners to realize how long the educational process can be.
    d. solidify the bond between learner and educator. ____

27. By supporting students' interaction in the classroom, educators have expanded a lifelong network of:
   a. clubs.
   b. interpersonal relationships.
   c. partners.
   d. none of the above. ____

28. When developing activities for learners, the master educator will offer choices in order to:
   a. confuse the learners.
   b. make the learners feel they have control.
   c. make the learners feel the educator is indecisive.
   d. cause anxiety in the learners. ____

29. Our overall appearance, our facial expressions, body language, posture, and gestures:
   a. represents 7 percent of the message we are delivering to our learners.
   b. represents 38 percent of the message we are delivering to our learners.
   c. represents 45 percent of the message we are delivering to our learners.
   d. represent 55 percent of the message we are delivering to our learners. ____

30. To challenge learners, the master educator will be:
   a. unenthusiastic.
   b. animated.
   c. dull.
   d. disinterested. ____

31. When delivering a presentation, the master educator will:
   a. be sincere and focus on learners.
   b. put the focus on the educator.
   c. worry about the presentation.
   d. be concerned with the teaching strategy. ____

32. To convey sincerity and interest throughout the presentation, the educator should:
   a. gaze at the walls.
   b. maintain eye contact with all learners throughout the presentation.
   c. stare at one student throughout the presentation.
   d. constantly look at the clock. ____

33. Learners like to know what is in store for them; thus, the master educator will:
   a. not preview the lesson.
   b. give a review at the end of the day.
   c. give students a general overview of the day's lesson at the beginning.
   d. tell only those who ask. ____

34. You convey visual integrity through:
   a. your articulation.
   b. vocabulary and higher-order thinking skills.
   c. verbal skills.
   d. appearance, facial expressions, posture, and body language. ____

35. The way you speak your message will impact your students; so, to have a positive outcome:
   a. speak clearly.
   b. speak pleasantly.
   c. speak without any affectations.
   d. all of the above. ____

36. Being able to speak clearly, distinctly, and in a manner in which everyone can understand is called:
   a. distinction.   **c.** pitch.
   b. articulation.   **d.** tonality. ____

37. When each sentence ensures a pleasant and friendly sound, we are varying the:
   a. tone.   **c.** articulation.
   b. pace.   **d.** pitch. ____

38. When stating key words that are important to the lesson, use:
   a. emphasis.
   b. a loud voice.
   c. a quiet voice so students have to strain to hear.
   d. none of the above. ____

39. Facial expressions often give a different quality to the meaning of your words; this is called:
   a. tone.   **c.** articulation.
   b. pace.   **d.** emphasis. ____

40. The vocabulary the master educator uses must:
    a. be appropriate for the learning level of the students.
    b. be pronounced properly.
    c. not be condescending.
    d. all of the above. ____

41. Master educators will use powerful openings to establish
    and maintain a sincere rapport with the learner. They will
    use the first:
    a. 35 minutes to inform and excite the learners.
    b. 25 minutes to inform and excite the learners.
    c. 15 minutes to inform and excite the learners.
    d. 5 minutes to inform and excite the learners. ____

42. The structure the educator might use in a situation that has
    caused a problem or concern is the:
    a. chronological structure.   c. spatial structure.
    b. problem/solution structure.   d. topical structure. ____

43. The structure that the educator would find appropriate when
    presenting the evolution of a service is the:
    a. chronological structure.
    b. problem/solution structure.
    c. topical structure.
    d. theory and practice structure. ____

44. The qualitative structure that allows you to list your points in
    the order of significance, with the most important discussed
    at the beginning of the lesson, when the learner's attention
    is sharpest, is called:
    a. topical.   c. spatial.
    b. problem/solution.   d. none of the above. ____

45. The structure that an educator might find helpful to begin
    an overview of general subject matter and progress to the
    specific, or vice versa, is the:
    a. topical structure.
    b. chronological structure.
    c. problem/solution structure.
    d. spatial structure. ____

46. The structure the educator uses to outline the theory of any given subject and then demonstrate how it works in practice is the:
    a. spatial structure.
    b. theory/practice structure.
    c. topical structure.
    d. problem/solution structure. ____

47. To add credibility to presentations, include information from:
    a. direct observation.
    b. quoted statistical information.
    c. verifiable sources.
    d. all of the choices. ____

48. Providing analogies to learners will:
    a. give the students something to think about.
    b. make a concept more understandable.
    c. allow students to develop higher-level thinking skills.
    d. none of the above. ____

49. The part of the lesson that includes a summary, restatement of key points, and performance for the learner is the:
    a. opening.   c. closing.
    b. body.   d. none of the above. ____

50. Closing the lesson with a powerful punch is achieved with:
    a. humor and poems.
    b. anecdotes.
    c. assessment and evaluation.
    d. all of the above. ____

51. The technique that master educators use to shift from one activity to another is called:
    a. transition.   c. turnover.
    b. shift.   d. none of the above. ____

52. A powerful strategy to move from one activity to another is to:
    a. use a pause and then move on.
    b. use silence and then move to the next activity.
    c. stand quietly for moment, indicating the next activity is ready to begin.
    d. all of the above. ____

53. Instructing learners to think about the material that has been presented and formulating questions is a helpful review as well as:
    a. a problem for some learners.
    b. a time-waster.
    c. a transition into the next part of the lesson.
    d. disruptive. ____

54. Adult learners can listen with understanding for:
    a. 90 minutes.
    b. 70 minutes.
    c. 50 minutes.
    d. 20 minutes. ____

55. Learners can only listen with retention of the information for:
    a. 90 minutes.
    b. 70 minutes.
    c. 50 minutes.
    d. 20 minutes. ____

56. The master educator will vary the stimuli every:
    a. 90 minutes.
    b. 70 minutes.
    c. 20 minutes.
    d. 15 minutes. ____

57. The master educator will use gestures to:
    a. lend emphasis.
    b. clarify meaning.
    c. help reveal the educator's attitudes.
    d. all of the above. ____

58. An energizer is an activity that gives learners a mental break, keeps them focused, and lasts:
    a. 1 to 3 minutes.
    b. 3 to 5 minutes.
    c. 5 to 8 minutes.
    d. 8 to 11 minutes. ____

59. The master educator will plan suitable questions:
    a. during the classroom presentation.
    b. prior to the classroom presentation.
    c. while waiting for the students to ask them.
    d. all of the above. ____

60. Master educators will formulate questions that:
    a. are simple.
    b. are to the point.
    c. make logical transitions between questions.
    d. all of the above. ____

61. The _____ questioning technique requires short
answers.
   a. low-order   **c.** high-order
   b. center-order   **d.** no-order   _____

62. Research shows that higher-level questioning may lead to
improved achievement for learners who have the following
abilities:
   a. comprehension.   **c.** information synthesis.
   b. data analysis.   **d.** all of the above.   _____

63. A method for questioning would be:
   a. direct questioning.
   b. indirect questioning.
   c. sinusoidal questioning.
   d. faradic questioning.   _____

64. When the educator questions a specific student and then
asks another student to comment on the first student's
response, the educator is using:
   a. group questioning.   **c.** indirect questioning.
   b. direct questioning.   **d.** redirect questioning.   _____

65. Effective listening is an important part of answering
questions. The master educator will listen to the emotion
behind the question, and:
   a. be responsive to all questions.
   b. restate the question for clarity.
   c. verify that the questioner has been satisfied by the
      answer.
   d. all of the above.   _____

CHAPTER 8 Effective Classroom Management and Supervision

MULTIPLE CHOICE

1. Master educators will provide an environment filled with motivation, energy, enthusiasm, and excitement because of their attitude of:
   - **a.** classroom decor.
   - **b.** decorum.
   - **c.** caring.
   - **d.** propriety. ____

2. To establish credibility and authority and to generate a high degree of cooperation in a teaching situation, the master educator must:
   - **a.** project a professional image.
   - **b.** be well groomed.
   - **c.** control the environment.
   - **d.** have good posture. ____

3. Classroom conflicts and misunderstandings may be avoided if the master educator:
   - **a.** is firm and demanding.
   - **b.** conducts class like a drill sergeant and is unwavering within the class environment.
   - **c.** sets well-defined guidelines and expectations for leaner behavior.
   - **d.** starts each day with new set of guidelines to follow. ____

4. Allowing students to develop the guidelines for professionalism within the classroom may:
   - **a.** cause chaos.
   - **b.** cause students to commit themselves to the standards they have developed.
   - **c.** result in conflicting standards.
   - **d.** cause more harm than good. ____

5. Behavior guidelines should be set forth in a specific document and should include:
   - **a.** consequences for noncompliance.
   - **b.** rules and standards.
   - **c.** performance objectives.
   - **d.** both a and b. ____

6. The appropriate time to discuss guidelines for behavior is:
   a. at the first visit to the institution.
   b. after the first infraction of a rule.
   c. in the new student orientation process.
   d. all of the above. ____

7. For the learner to learn, the master educator must facilitate the learning process through:
   a. the maintenance of high behavioral standards.
   b. consistency in enforcing rules and applying consequences.
   c. modeling appropriate conduct.
   d. all of the above. ____

8. Desired behaviors will be achieved more readily if the master educator reacts:
   a. positively.   c. quickly.
   b. negatively.   d. sarcastically. ____

9. All misconduct cannot be eliminated, but master educators will model and teach students to:
   a. develop self-control.   c. use ridicule.
   b. develop hostility.   d. use sarcasm. ____

10. Using the least amount of force necessary to control misbehavior is termed:
    a. minimal consequences.
    b. low-profile intervention.
    c. maximum intervention.
    d. low-proximity response. ____

11. Behaving the same way on repeated occasions when the circumstances are the same or similar is termed:
    a. uniformity.   c. regularity.
    b. consistency.   d. harmony. ____

12. The state or quality of acting the same or with the same standard among different parties or learners is called:
    a. consistency.   c. compatibility.
    b. uniformity.   d. harmony. ____

13. Surveys indicate that inconsistent application of policies and procedures among learners:
   a. is of no concern.
   b. causes conflicting messages.
   c. is of significant concern.
   d. both b and c.   ____

14. The method of dealing with misconduct that is very direct and assertive is termed:
   a. close-proximity intervention.
   b. low-profile intervention.
   c. high-profile intervention.
   d. assertive discipline.   ____

15. When selecting a method of controlling misconduct, the master educator should:
   a. stick to one method.
   b. become familiar with a variety of methods and choose accordingly.
   c. use low-profile intervention.
   d. use high-profile intervention.   ____

16. Being dignified in behavior, speech, and dress is called:
   a. professionalism.   c. dignity.
   b. decorum.   d. grooming.   ____

17. Misbehavior is better managed if the educator maintains decorum and:
   a. proper vocabulary.
   b. continuity and inconsistency.
   c. a high degree of professionalism.
   d. eye contact.   ____

18. Ignoring a student's behavior may be an acceptable strategy if the misconduct is:
   a. insignificant.   c. chronic.
   b. hostile.   d. disruptive.   ____

19. During a presentation or group discussion, the educator might insert the name of the learner in an instructional statement; this strategy is known as:
   a. naming names.
   b. name-dropping.
   c. reclaiming the disruptive student.
   d. stopping the chatterbox.   ____

20. Physically moving toward the learner is a powerful means of controlling a misbehavior; the term for this strategy is:
   a. proximity stroll.
   b. stand by me.
   c. close proximity.
   d. parallel parking. ____

21. When using a verbal desist, it is very important not to attack the character of the learner, but to:
   a. speak angrily.
   b. convey hostility.
   c. become sarcastic.
   d. address the situation. ____

22. When selecting remedies for misconduct, the educator considers:
   a. school policies.
   b. the nature of the misconduct.
   c. the personal style of the educator.
   d. all of the above. ____

23. Reprimands are one of the most common remedial techniques; they should occur as soon after the misbehavior as possible. If a resolution to the problem is expected, there must be:
   a. rules and consequences.
   b. punishments with suspensions.
   c. clarification and caring.
   d. contracts for better behavior. ____

24. A document stating the arrangement made between the educator and the learner regarding a greater commitment toward agreed-upon behavior is called a(n):
   a. agreement or contract.
   b. statement of purpose.
   c. will of intent.
   d. promissory note. ____

25. When planning for a behavioral conference, the educator should consider:
   a. specific areas of documented misconduct.
   b. concrete goals for improvement.
   c. consequences for failure to remedy misconduct.
   d. all of the above. ____

26. Counseling services and advice to learners on areas of employment, licensing, professional assistance, and reciprocity are required by many state regulatory agencies and accrediting bodies; this service is termed:
    a. academic advisement.
    b. public relations.
    c. professional development.
    d. professional services.   ____

27. Through academic advisement a student may review progress through a program of study and establish:
    a. loyalty, decorum, and positive affirmations.
    b. approval, recognition, and appreciation.
    c. recognition and appreciation.
    d. approval and appreciation.   ____

9 Achieving Learner Results

MULTIPLE CHOICE

1. The Americans with Disabilities Act protects those Americans who are physically or mentally impaired, such as:
   a. those engaged in the illegal use of drugs.
   b. those with orthodontics.
   c. those who have substantial limitations in one or more "major life activities."
   d. those needing eye glasses. ____

2. The agency that prohibits discrimination on the basis of disability in both public and private sectors is:
   a. FERPA.
   b. OSHA.
   c. EPA.
   d. ADA. ____

3. Title III of the American with Disabilities Act defines "readily achievable" as:
   a. can be easily accomplished and carried out without much difficulty or expense.
   b. can be mastered by the individual without much difficulty or effort.
   c. the task the client performs is made under the same conditions without any alterations.
   d. all of the above. ____

4. Schools with people with disabilities must ensure to:
   a. furnish auxiliary aids when necessary to ensure effective communication, unless undue burden or fundamental alteration would result.
   b. eliminate unnecessary eligibility standards or rules that deny individuals with disabilities an equal opportunity to enjoy the goods and services of the place of accommodation.
   c. provide reasonable modification in policies, practices, and procedures that deny equal access to individuals.
   d. all of the above. ____

5. Modifications to institutions made in accordance with ADA could include:
   a. permitting extended time for course completion.
   b. providing auxiliary aids or services.
   c. permitting the course to be completed in a more accessible location or making alternative arrangements.
   d. all of the above. ____

6. Proof of disability rests on:
   a. the institution enrolling the student.
   b. the disabled person who desires to enroll in the postsecondary school.
   c. the ADA.
   d. the oversight agency. ____

7. The individual accommodation plan for the disabled learner is the responsibility of the:
   a. institution that enrolls the learner.
   b. learner with a disability choosing the program.
   c. ADA.
   d. oversight agency. ____

8. The accommodation plan might include:
   a. textbooks on tape.
   b. seeing-eye canine.
   c. removal of a wall in the school.
   d. the raising of the ceiling. ____

9. In North America the term *learning disability* refers to:
   a. low intelligence levels.
   b. the absence of information on an intellectual level.
   c. a group of disorders that affect a broad range of academic and functional skills.
   d. the lack of mental activity and a diminished capacity for learning. ____

10. The brain processes information in four ways; the information perceived through the senses, such as visual and auditory perception, is referred to as:
    a. input.   c. storage.
    b. integration.   d. output. ____

11. Information comes from the brain either through words or through muscle activity, such as gesturing, writing, or drawing. This stage of information processing is referred to as:
    a. input.
    b. integration.
    c. storage.
    d. output.   ____

12. The stage in which perceived input is interpreted, categorized, placed in a sequence, or related to previous learning is called:
    a. input.
    b. integration.
    c. storage.
    d. output.   ____

13. Answering a question on demand and putting thoughts into words before we speak is an information process called:
    a. input.
    b. integration.
    c. storage.
    d. output.   ____

14. Most memory difficulties occur in the area of short-term memory, which can make it difficult to learn new material without many more repetitions that usual; this problem affects information
    a. input.
    b. integration.
    c. storage.
    d. output.   ____

15. Dyslexia is a specific learning disability that hinders the learning of our students and is:
    a. neurologically based.
    b. congenital.
    c. a developmental condition.
    d. all of the above.   ____

16. The cause of dyslexia:
    a. has not been confirmed.
    b. is the use of cell phones.
    c. is the administration of the polio vaccine.
    d. is the administration of the rubella vaccine.   ____

17. The dyslexic learner may act out by displaying characteristics that:
    a. demonstrate effective listening.
    b. demonstrate carelessness.
    c. give the appearance of concentration.
    d. are graceful.   ____

18. It is encouraging to find that dyslexic learners:
   a. have a good visual eye.
   b. are imaginative.
   c. are skillful with their hands.
   d. all of the above. ____

19. When teaching the dyslexic learner, the master educator should:
   a. review the learner's past academic file if available.
   b. understand the student's specific difficulties.
   c. gain an understanding of the student's learning style.
   d. all of the above. ____

20. Master educators will assist the dyslexic learner with:
   a. time management.   **c.** sequencing.
   b. organization.   **d.** all of the above. ____

21. Various teaching strategies should be utilized with the dyslexic learner, along with:
   a. peer coaching.
   b. workbook activities.
   c. silent reading.
   d. textbook outlining. ____

22. Since the dyslexic learner learns best through hands-on experience, demonstrations, experimentation, observation, and visual aids, educators should use:
   a. straight outline form.
   b. copying of material from the overhead or board.
   c. reading aloud by students.
   d. multisensory methods for practicing and learning. ____

23. Master educators should remember that the dyslexic learner:
   a. may have difficulty with figures.
   b. may be personally disorganized.
   c. has difficulty taking notes.
   d. all of the above. ____

24. Attention deficit hyperactivity disorder is defined by the American Academy of Pediatrics as:
    a. a chronic neurological dysfunction within the central nervous system that is not related to gender, level of intelligence, or cultural environment.
    b. a rare nervous disorder that results from nerve damage caused by the body's own defenses, usually in response to an infection or other illness. This causes muscle weakness, loss of reflexes, and numbness or tingling in the arms, legs, face, and other parts of the body.
    c. a brain disorder that often interferes with a person's ability to communicate with and relate to others. Different areas of the brain fail to work together.
    d. a lower level of serotonin, a brain chemical, in the winter. ____

25. The cause of ADHD is still unknown, although some environmental factors affect it, including:
    a. diet and certain medications.
    b. parenting techniques.
    c. in some cases, artificial color and certain foods.
    d. all of the above. ____

26. ADHD learners have problems staying on required tasks, especially if they are not interested in the subject matter; such learners may:
    a. be easily distracted.
    b. be forgetful in daily activities.
    c. not seem to listen when spoken to directly.
    d. all of the above. ____

27. When ADHD learners find it difficult to stay on task, often act before thinking, act as if "driven by a motor," and talk excessively, they are displaying:
    a. impulsivity.   c. hyperactivity.
    b. inconsistency.   d. attentiveness. ____

28. There are a number of symptoms the educator can watch for to determine if a student has ADHD:
    a. confused by letters, numbers, and words.
    b. problems staying on required tasks, especially if they are not interested in the subject matter.
    c. difficulty putting thoughts into words; transposes phrases.
    d. has trouble writing or copying; hand writing is illegible. ____

29. Because the student with ADHD may be overwhelmed by too much stimulation, the master educator will:
    a. encourage the learner to persevere.
    b. help to build self-esteem.
    c. provide various teaching strategies to capture the attention of the learner.
    d. all of the above. ____

30. Which of the following strategies may prove beneficial to ADHD learners?
    a. Provide learners a quiet area without distraction when testing or studying.
    b. Provide instructions both in writing and orally.
    c. Allow sufficient time for the learner to thoughtfully prepare answers.
    d. All of the above. ____

31. Strategies that will support ADHD learners include:
    a. hand-write tests and outlines for the learners.
    b. divide projects and assignments into page-long segments.
    c. give them room to move about and release excess energy.
    d. use outdated videos to interest the learners. ____

32. Other strategies for ADHD learners include:
    a. develop a system of discreet "cues" that will alert learners in advance that you are going to call on them.
    b. give practice quizzes prior to the official test.
    c. consider alternative testing methods that will also demonstrate what the student has learned.
    d. all of the above. ____

33. We have learned that an effective second sensory-motor activity, such as tapping a pencil or clicking a pen, helps the learner stay alert; the master educator can facilitate a more positive activity that does not distract other, such as:
    a. using a clicker or timers.
    b. use of colored scented markers.
    c. use of stress balls.
    d. all of the above. ____

34. It is beneficial for educators to recognize chronic behavior such as:
   a. attention to detail.
   b. poor motivation and lack of interest.
   c. perfect attendance.
   d. good self-esteem.   ____

35. Persons with substance abuse problems are protected by the ADA and should be:
   a. referred to the appropriate professional source for help.
   b. given "reasonable accommodations.".
   c. subject to the same documentation standards as other students with disabilities.
   d. all of the above.   ____

36. To make the student more comfortable in the classroom, the master educator will:
   a. talk down to the learner.
   b. evaluate the learner at every opportunity.
   c. encourage self-confidence.
   d. treat the adult learner as a child.   ____

37. Knowing the barriers to learning will prove to be an asset to the educator; be on the alert for:
   a. learner apprehension.
   b. rapid response.
   c. lack of learner motivation.
   d. all of the above.   ____

38. Students exhibiting anxiety in the classroom need the educator to:
   a. be empathetic.   c. be illogical.
   b. be indifferent.   d. be inconsistent.   ____

39. Apprehensive students will compare themselves, their knowledge, and their responses to the way they are perceived by everyone else in the classroom; thus, the master educator will:
   a. establish a competitive classroom.
   b. establish strong and frequent eye contact.
   c. have the learner speak before the group.
   d. all of the above.   ____

40. Master educators use memory cues known as:
    a. game maps.
    b. puzzles.
    c. mnemonics.
    d. mind maps.   ____

41. Older learners may feel that they don't remember things
    as well as they did when they were younger; the master
    educator will aid in:
    a. providing distractions.
    b. increasing noise activity.
    c. providing uncomfortable work areas.
    d. creating a safe learning environment.   ____

42. Sometimes learners respond too quickly; to overcome this
    barrier to learning, the master educator will provide:
    a. speed in practical skills.
    b. opportunities for self-pacing.
    c. no opportunity for learners to respond immediately.
    d. all of the above.   ____

43. When the learner simply does not want to be in class, the
    educator will incorporate:
    a. ice-breakers and motivational tactics.
    b. various texts.
    c. workbook activities.
    d. journal activities.   ____

44. Many barriers to education may be created by the
    behaviors and attitudes of the:
    a. administrators.
    b. educators.
    c. students.
    d. clients.   ____

45. Learners are placed in an active learning mood by:
    a. using video.
    b. using computers.
    c. varying the teaching stimuli.
    d. using PowerPoint.   ____

46. A conducive environment for learning would include:
    a. questions are encouraged.
    b. avoidance of eye contact.
    c. boring lectures.
    d. uncomfortable temperature.   ____

47. By encouraging interpersonal relationships among learners, the master educator expands their:
    a. circle of friends.
    b. perimeter.
    c. association.
    d. network. ____

48. To support the content of classes and show learners how information will work for them:
    a. talk about what you are trying to teach.
    b. use examples and illustrations.
    c. use the textbook.
    d. use the workbook. ____

49. The master educator will take personal steps to become knowledgeable about all learning disabilities or disorders and come to the realization that:
    a. learner behavior or performance may not meet the standards we have established for other learners.
    b. the learner may have difficulty sustaining attention to tasks due to poor motivation.
    c. the learners' poor performance is due to laziness or other internal characteristics.
    d. the learner blurts out because of rudeness. ____

50. When working with a dyslexic learner, the master educator may find:
    a. there is inadequate storage of knowledge.
    b. poor memory skills.
    c. there may be inadequate vocabulary.
    d. all of the above. ____

CHAPTER 10
Program Review, Development, and Lesson Planning

MULTIPLE CHOICE

1. The curriculum development process includes:
   a. identifying units of instruction prescribed by any applicable oversight agency.
   b. defining and allocating learning outcomes for students.
   c. developing lesson plans and a systematic method of student evaluation.
   d. all of the above.   ____

2. When developing a program of study, you will be directed by:
   a. documents and textbooks available.
   b. state regulatory agencies.
   c. professional associations.
   d. all of the above.   ____

3. When developing the curriculum, you will also:
   a. review the information obtained.
   b. list essential tasks and topics.
   c. sort the topics and tasks.
   d. all of the above.   ____

4. One way to sequence the subject categories is:
   a. by the order in which tasks are performed within the occupation.
   b. from the most basic to the most complex.
   c. from general to more specific subject matter.
   d. all of the above.   ____

5. When allocating time for each subject in your curriculum, be guided by:
   a. regulatory oversight agencies.
   b. clinic regulations.
   c. professional associations.
   d. federal guidelines.   ____

6. Units of instruction will concentrate on:
   a. topics within each category.
   b. one or a few topics within the subject.
   c. many topics within the subject.
   d. none of the above.   ____

7. A comprehensive and organized written plan of instruction that includes the program description, topics to be taught, learning goals and objectives, resources, and other material pertinent for delivery of a cosmetology program is a:
   a. learning guide.
   b. state standard.
   c. program outline.
   d. performance guideline. _____

8. Master educators who have been teaching for a long time find lesson planning invaluable because:
   a. it ensures that students receive detailed information.
   b. it has been a long time since they have been in the salon as working stylists.
   c. they have gotten older and long-term memory is failing.
   d. none of the above. _____

9. Developing a comprehensive schedule is vital to ensure that:
   a. students meet hour requirements.
   b. lessons can be completed in the time allocated.
   c. students are able to take extended vacations.
   d. none of the above. _____

10. A(n) _____ includes information about the educational program, a detailed program syllabus and description of the program's elements, school policies and procedures, and other general information that will further assist in the success of the student.
    a. orientation program
    b. educational planning program
    c. program planning initiative
    d. introduction and indoctrination program _____

11. An institution's advisory council can bring help and resources to assist the institution:
    a. in identifying skills that need to be taught.
    b. by bringing their own experiences and resources.
    c. in prioritizing subject matter.
    d. all of the above. _____

12. The institution's advisory council is generally comprised of:
    a. school owners and directors.
    b. educators.
    c. employers within the applicable field of study.
    d. all of the above. _____

13. Maximum learning and retention by the students will be secured when the subjects and tasks have been:
    a. organized and sequenced in a logical manner.
    b. written in a format that is easily read by all students.
    c. organized in a manner that is easy to handle and not heavy.
    d. reviewed. ____

14. The acquisition of knowledge such as demonstration of feelings, attitudes, or sensitivities toward other people, ideas, or things is known as the:
    a. affective domain of instructional outcomes.
    b. melancholia domain of instructional outcomes.
    c. cognitive domain of instructional outcomes.
    d. psychomotor domain of instructional outcomes. ____

15. Skill development as it relates to performance, which requires tools, objects, supplies, and equipment, is the:
    a. affective domain of instructional outcomes.
    b. melancholia domain of instructional outcomes.
    c. cognitive domain of instructional outcomes.
    d. psychomotor domain of instructional outcomes. ____

16. Employers wish to hire people who have positive attitudes, get along well with fellow workers, possess a good work ethic, and are happy in their profession, qualities which relate to the:
    a. cognitive domain of instructional outcomes.
    b. melancholia domain of instructional outcomes.
    c. affective domain of instructional outcomes.
    d. psychomotor domain of instructional outcomes. ____

17. The master educator will make the lesson objectives:
    a. difficult.   c. measurable.
    b. complex.   d. easy to master. ____

18. For objectives to be clear, the master educator will state:
    a. how the activity will be measured.
    b. the desired performance.
    c. the conditions of the learning activity.
    d. all of the above. ____

19. In the assessment process, the master educator will recognize that treating all students alike is:
    a. appropriate.
    b. inappropriate.
    c. a good teaching method.
    d. fair and equitable. ____

20. The goal of the educator is to have the graduates:
    a. draw conclusions about what they observe.
    b. think critically and creatively.
    c. analyze situations.
    d. all of the above. ____

21. The program outline will generally contain:
    a. names and addresses of students.
    b. student social security numbers.
    c. the educator's home address.
    d. none of the above. ____

22. Contained in the program outline are:
    a. instructional methods.
    b. grading procedures.
    c. learning goals and objectives.
    d. all of the above. ____

23. A comprehensive library will include:
    a. picture books.
    b. games for downtime.
    c. references, periodicals, and audio/videotapes.
    d. lounge chairs. ____

24. Providing education through a sequential set of learning units that may be necessary for state board preparation is called:
    a. units of instruction.   c. block schedules.
    b. clock-hour education.   d. credits. ____

25. When evaluating practical assignments, use procedure and performance standards:
    a. in the Practical Cosmetology Skills Competency Evaluation Criteria.
    b. established by the state licensing agency.
    c. according to the text procedures.
    d. all of the above. ____

26. Practical skill assignments rated:
    a. completed are counted toward program completion.
    b. satisfactory or better are counted toward program completion.
    c. attempted are counted toward program completion.
    d. excused because of absence are counted toward program completion. ____

27. The best opportunity to review policies, procedures, and consumer information required by accrediting and federal agencies is:
    a. at break time a little each day.
    b. individually with each student.
    c. at back-to-school night.
    d. at new student orientation before the first day or on the first day. ____

28. A comprehensive orientation program should be organized within:
    a. a box.
    b. a thee-ring binder.
    c. separate folders.
    d. plastic sheet protectors. ____

29. The perfect time to have students sign off as to having received information required by state regulatory and accrediting agencies is:
    a. during clinic time.
    b. at break.
    c. at orientation.
    d. during class time. ____

30. An activity that allows new students to bond with continuing students is a(n):
    a. word search.
    b. workbook assignment.
    c. crossword puzzle.
    d. ice-breaker. ____

31. The orientation program is a new beginning for the learner; thus it would be appropriate for the educator to:
    a. introduce all staff.
    b. introduce only admissions representatives.
    c. introduce the school owner only.
    d. introduce the counselor only. ____

32. The _____ explains how the learner's progress and attendance might affect the program of training.
    a. school owner
    b. financial aid officer
    c. counselor
    d. educator ____

33. The outward reflection of inner feelings, thoughts, attitudes, and values defines:
    a. character.
    b. personality.
    c. dignity.
    d. temperament. ____

34. A "just for laughs" ungraded orientation quiz can be given to determine:
    a. if review is necessary.
    b. if more clarification is needed.
    c. retention of important information.
    d. all of the above. ____

35. The master educator will plan lessons that are:
    a. individualized.
    b. clearly written.
    c. flexible.
    d. all of the above. ____

36. All lesson plans should be based on the needs, interests, and:
    a. likes of the students.
    b. feelings of the students.
    c. abilities of the students.
    d. choices of the students. ____

37. Lesson plans are based on the:
    a. goals of the individual educator.
    b. needs of the individual educator.
    c. goals of the learner.
    d. style of the individual educator. ____

38. In order to be effective, lesson plans will:
    a. stay the same; there is no need to change them when the underlying theory is the same.
    b. be adhered to in the fashion of the previous educators; if it worked for them it will work for us.
    c. change as today's learner changes; they need to be changed and updated frequently to deliver the most current information.
    d. none of the above. ____

39. One advantage of having a lesson plan is that:
    a. older students could take over your class.
    b. you could copy it and give it to the students for notes.
    c. learners have the benefit of appropriate summarization and review.
    d. substitute teachers could use it. ____

40. Upon reading the lesson objective, the learner should have:
    a. a clear understanding of what is to be accomplished.
    b. some idea of what is expected.
    c. further need of explanation.
    d. peer coaching to assist in understanding of the objective. ____

41. A lesson objective dealing with the affective domain deals with:
    a. the arts.
    b. skill development.
    c. the acquisition of knowledge.
    d. people skills. ____

42. By listing implements, materials, and equipment needed to deliver the lesson, the educator can:
    a. deliver an orderly and organized lesson.
    b. begin the class on time.
    c. notify the class ahead of time of what will be needed.
    d. all of the above. ____

43. When using audiovisual equipment, the educator must:
    a. see that it is operational and available for class.
    b. check it out just before class.
    c. preview the video with the class.
    d. set up the equipment with the class in the room. ____

44. Time allocated for each lesson should be listed on the educator's plan; allocated time may vary because of:
    a. unscheduled breaks.
    b. class not starting on time.
    c. the number of activities in the lesson.
    d. a student having a flat tire. ____

45. Having the student read a topic before the class is given as the component of the lesson plan called:
    a. notes.   c. educational aids.
    b. prior student assignment.   d. homework. ____

46. Lessons that have reinforcement ideas, reminders, and perhaps inspirational thoughts for the day included are called:
    a. tips for the teacher.   c. notes to the educator.
    b. comments for the teacher.   d. notes. ____

47. The introduction of the lesson will consist of:
    a. a review of prior learning.
    b. a statement of concern.
    c. reasons for using certain products.
    d. how the supplies will be distributed. ____

48. In order to gain the interest of the students before entering the classroom, and continuing throughout the day, the master educator will set a process in motion that will motivate the learner. This process is called:
    a. motivational moments.   c. the anticipatory set.
    b. the hook.   d. I've gotcha. ____

49. The educator notes for the presentation outline should be:
    a. comprehensive, organized, and properly sequenced.
    b. written so that only the educator understands them.
    c. filled with markings.
    d. brief and to the point. ____

50. To retain the interest of the learner, educators must vary the stimuli for students at least every:
    a. two minutes.   c. six minutes.
    b. four minutes.   d. eight minutes. ____

11 Educational Aids and Technology in the Classroom

MULTIPLE CHOICE

1. Instructional aids will support:
   a. learning resources.
   b. technology.
   c. creative teaching methods.
   d. none of the above. ____

2. To maintain student interest the educator will:
   a. use video presentations often.
   b. vary instructional materials.
   c. make use of workbook assignments.
   d. encourage students to take notes. ____

3. Instructional aids provide for a change of pace and also:
   a. clarify information.
   b. provide busy time.
   c. give educators time to collaborate.
   d. give students time to catch up on work. ____

4. Learners often place more emphasis on what they:
   a. hear.   c. feel.
   b. touch.   d. see. ____

5. Learners think at a rate of:
   a. 110 to 200 words per minute.
   b. 200 to 300 words per minute.
   c. 300 to 400 words per minute.
   d. 400 to 500 words per minute. ____

6. When the educator addresses more of the learners' senses during a presentation, there is a greater opportunity for:
   a. understanding and retention.   c. agitation.
   b. confusion.   d. perplexity. ____

7. Clear visual aids may be used to:
   a. give directions.
   b. clear up misinformation.
   c. increase comprehension.
   d. all of the above. ____

8. By adding visual aids to the spoken message, learners will:
   a. hear more and retain more.
   b. use all of their senses.
   c. gain the information more quickly, reducing required presentation time.
   d. gain the information through their most dominant learning style. ____

9. Bringing the salon environment into the classroom with PowerPoint presentations, pictures, and so forth adds:
   a. a diversion.
   b. a real-world perspective.
   c. another teaching skill.
   d. dimension. ____

10. By using more visual aids in the presentation of the lesson, the educator can be more confident and:
    a. ensure consistency.
    b. diminish comprehension.
    c. obscure visibility.
    d. exert authority. ____

11. With today's diverse student population, it is the responsibility of the educator to:
    a. assign homework that is not time-consuming.
    b. speak several languages.
    c. use a variety of teaching materials.
    d. find someone who can translate other languages. ____

12. Important concepts for selecting and preparing a visual aid include:
    a. visibility.
    b. clarification.
    c. proportion.
    d. all of the above. ____

13. Instructional materials that are standard print materials (nonprojected) are used for:
    a. flip charts.
    b. visuals during a presentation.
    c. reference.
    d. all of the above. ____

14. Workbooks are written to complement and support the textbook; the major advantage of the workbook is that:
    a. students can use it independently.
    b. it fills in downtime.
    c. it can be used as a consequence for misbehavior.
    d. when it is totally completed the student can graduate. ____

15. Information that is more current than that contained in the textbook may be found in:
    a. trade journal articles.
    b. industry periodicals.
    c. newspaper articles.
    d. all of the above. ____

16. Career opportunities in the United States can be found in the:
    a. Occupational Possibility Handbook.
    b. Occupational Outlook Handbook.
    c. Occupational Prospect Handbook.
    d. Occupational Opportunity Handbook. ____

17. A key component in self-study or self-instructional systems, and also an asset to the slower learner who needs repetition for maximum retention, are:
    a. reference books.
    b. workbooks.
    c. audiotapes or CD-ROMs.
    d. flip charts. ____

18. Visual presentation can increase retention, enhance learning, and make effective use of instructional time. In order to accomplish this, the tools:
    a. should be kept simple.
    b. should have materials properly attached.
    c. should make use of digital cameras.
    d. all of the above. ____

19. The white magnetic marker board or multipurpose board may be used with:
    a. magic markers.   c. special marking pens.
    b. colored chalk.   d. crayons. ____

20. When using the chalkboard or the magnetic board, the educator:
    a. must speak to the learners, not to the board.
    b. must always begin with a clean board.
    c. should use printed letters rather than script.
    d. all of the above. ____

21. Flip charts are suitable for groups no larger than:
    a. 40.   c. 50.
    b. 45.   d. 55. ____

22. Flip charts are useful in illustrating sequential steps in a process as long as the educator:
    a. places each major step on a single sheet.
    b. lists the steps on one sheet.
    c. uses half of a page for each step.
    d. none of the above. ____

23. The type of projector that enables you to project solid images onto a surface to diagram is the:
    a. laser disc.
    c. LCD projector.
    b. overhead projector.
    d. opaque projector. ____

24. One of the most common, flexible, and economical instructional tools used in the classroom is the:
    a. overhead projector.
    c. opaque projector.
    b. LCD projector.
    d. white magnetic board. ____

25. The best thing about working with transparencies is:
    a. you face the class while writing the material on the film.
    b. they work well when the room is well lit.
    c. they can be prepared ahead of time.
    d. all of the above. ____

26. One disadvantage to using transparencies is:
    a. the bulb may burn out when in the middle of a lesson.
    b. commercially prepared versions are available.
    c. they are easy for students to see.
    d. you are facing away from students while writing on them. ____

27. The master educator can produce professional-looking transparencies using:
    a. colored markers.
    b. felt marking crayons.
    c. desktop-type publishing software.
    d. colored chalk. ____

28. Incompatible film run through a copier will:
    a. tear the transparency.
    b. leave no imprint.
    c. melt the film inside the copier, causing an expensive repair.
    d. cause the film to be ruined. ____

29. Disadvantages in using the transparency include:
    a. no audio.
    c. classroom size.
    b. incorrect lighting.
    d. all of the above. ____

30. Using cartoons, charts, and illustrations in transparencies will:
    a. distract from the meaning.
    b. show that the content is not important.
    c. demonstrate that the educator is not serious.
    d. help to convey your meaning. ____

31. To provide maximum visibility, transparency lettering should be at least:
    a. 8-point typeface
    b. 18-point typeface.
    c. 28-point typeface.
    d. 38-point typeface.   ____

32. When drawing attention to a specific fact on the transparency:
    a. use a pointer as you would with a chalkboard.
    b. go up to the screen and point.
    c. don't use anything.
    d. use a laser pointer.   ____

33. Computer software has made education in this century:
    a. a source for independent study.
    b. too complex.
    c. complicated.
    d. much too expensive.   ____

34. The LCD projector allows images to be projected on a(n):
    a. television.
    b. overhead.
    c. large screen.
    d. monitor.   ____

35. When purchasing a LCD projector, consider:
    a. resolution and weight.
    b. brightness and contrast.
    c. connectivity and lamp life.
    d. all of the above.   ____

36. DVDs have a much higher capacity for storage; these devices have replaced:
    a. filmstrips.
    b. films.
    c. videos.
    d. all of the above.   ____

37. When considering the use of a video for a lesson, the educator will consider:
    a. how much time the video will free up for the educator.
    b. the people in the video.
    c. how the video address the learning objective.
    d. all of the above.   ____

38. Video presentations are not free time for students or educators; be certain:
    a. that learners know what they are expected to learn from the video.
    b. to become familiar with the content of the video.
    c. to prepare discussion questions for use before and after viewing of the video.
    d. all of the above.   ____

39. Students watching a video should:
   a. take elaborate notes.
   b. highlight the corresponding information in their textbooks.
   c. look through trade journals to find information on the topic.
   d. none of the above. _____

40. Key points should be introduced to the students:
   a. after the video.
   b. on a handout given during the video.
   c. before the video.
   d. on a handout given after the video. _____

41. Show the video a second time:
   a. whenever possible.
   b. immediately after the discussion.
   c. as a review at the beginning of the next class.
   d. all of the above. _____

42. When the video is presenting a technical procedure, the learners should:
   a. demonstrate the actual skills involved.
   b. list the procedures demonstrated in the video presentation.
   c. complete a crossword puzzle on the video presentation.
   d. outline the main components of the video presentation. _____

43. To determine the size of a television monitor for a classroom, plan for one diagonal inch of viewing screen for each student; thus, for a class of 25 you would want:
   a. two 19-inch monitors.   **c.** a 32-inch monitor.
   b. a 25-inch monitor.   **d.** a wide-screen monitor. _____

44. Master educators must recognize that distance learning is here to stay, but:
   a. it is not for the irresponsible learner.
   b. it will not replace hands-on learning.
   c. the educator can never be replaced.
   d. all of the above.

45. Social media and blogging about the class can cause students to:
   a. ignore friends and family who text them.
   b. become more invested in the topic.
   c. ignore school and skip classes.
   d. become less invested in the topic. ____

46. In today's classrooms it is necessary for educators to:
   a. know how to operate the equipment only.
   b. just use overhead projectors.
   c. know how to operate and maintain equipment effectively and safely.
   d. none of the above. ____

47. The master educator must be knowledgeable and skilled in the use of tools and equipment that will be used by the students, and must also teach student instructors:
   a. basic skills.
   b. advanced skills.
   c. salon procedures.
   d. intelligent decisions concerning purchase and maintenance of equipment. ____

48. When dealing with instructional equipment, it is imperative that it is:
   a. inspected.
   b. functioning according to the standards for quality education.
   c. operational.
   d. all of the above. ____

49. The master educator can plan for regular use of a variety of electronic teaching aids, such as:
   a. bulletin boards.   **c.** white boards.
   b. flip charts.   **d.** transparencies. ____

50. When setting up the viewing screen, it should be at least:
   a. 22 inches from the floor, which will allow most learners to see the full screen clearly.
   b. 32 inches from the floor, which will allow most learners to see the full screen clearly.
   c. 42 inches from the floor, which will allow most learners to see the full screen clearly.
   d. 52 inches from the floor, which will allow most learners to see the full screen clearly. ____

12 Assessing Progress and Advising Students

MULTIPLE CHOICE

1. Grading must correlate with:
   a. educational objectives.
   b. questioning techniques.
   c. the problem/solution structure.
   d. the topical structure. ____

2. The three main categories assessed and graded in schools of cosmetology and related career fields are theoretical knowledge, practical skills development, and:
   a. honesty and good grooming.
   b. loyalty and faithfulness.
   c. attitude and professionalism.
   d. wisdom and courage. ____

3. Practical assignments are evaluated as completed and counted toward course completion only when:
   a. they are completed.
   b. they are completed and rated as satisfactory or better.
   c. they are attempted.
   d. all of the above. ____

4. Students must maintain a minimum theory grade average of:
   a. 60 percent.   c. 70 percent.
   b. 65 percent.   d. 75 percent. ____

5. The learner's theoretical knowledge is usually assessed through written testing consisting of:
   a. true/false questions.
   b. multiple-choice questions.
   c. fill-in-the-blank questions.
   d. all of the above. ____

6. Practical skills and attitude are generally assessed using a performance evaluation method such as:
   a. action lists.   c. Likert scales.
   b. weighting scales.   d. red scales. ____

7. The evaluation that determines what the student knows after having been taught certain material or skills is called:
   a. scientific evaluation.
   c. revolving evaluation.
   b. outcome evaluation.
   d. preserving evaluation. ____

8. The process of assigning grades at established checkpoints or after a unit of study is termed:
   a. fulfillment evaluation.
   c. completing evaluation.
   b. conclusive evaluation.
   d. summative evaluation. ____

9. When grading, an important factor to consider is:
   a. consistency.
   c. failures.
   b. personal feeling.
   d. favoritism. ____

10. When grading, the educator must be:
    a. fair.
    c. honest.
    b. just.
    d. all of the above. ____

11. When educators ignore the predetermined performance criteria and grade according to their disposition, either good or bad, this is termed:
    a. grading by attitude.
    b. grading by emotion.
    c. grading by temperament.
    d. grading by disposition. ____

12. When an educator takes a personal dislike to a student and grades unfairly, it is harmful to the student's progress and self-esteem and is called:
    a. grading with delight.
    c. grading with spite.
    b. grading with pleasure.
    d. grading with rapture. ____

13. When the educator feels "it's my way or the highway," the educator is:
    a. grading by desire.
    c. grading by impulse.
    b. grading by personal fetish.
    d. grading with spite. ____

14. An educator who always gives an average grade, right in the middle, is:
    a. grading without risk.
    c. grading with a rubric.
    b. grading on a curve.
    d. grading with intention. ____

15. Learners will not have a clear understanding of how they are performing if the educator is:
    a. grading by attitude.
    c. grading without risk.
    b. grading by desire.
    d. none of the above. ____

16. Using a learner's past performance to measure the present is:
    a. grading by past experience.   **c.** grading by repetition.
    b. grading by assumption.   **d.** grading by supposition. ____

17. When the educator gets distracted, fails to see the end results of all services, and then sits down at the end of the day and simply writes grades for the students, the educator is:
    a. grading fairly.
    b. grading *in absentia.*
    c. grading with preoccupation.
    d. grading selectively. ____

18. The teacher who gives all students high grades is giving them a false perception of their skills and is:
    a. grading with TLC.
    b. grading with warm fuzzies.
    c. grading with faith, hope, and charity.
    d. grading with pity. ____

19. An outline of the content that will be covered by the test is called the:
    a. test plan.   **c.** test outline.
    b. rough draft.   **d.** teacher's test copy. ____

20. Tests that can be completed by at least 80 percent of the students within one hour are called:
    a. timed tests.   **c.** power tests.
    b. unit tests.   **d.** achievement tests. ____

21. In a true/false test, the student who has no prior knowledge of the subject has a:
    a. poor chance of selecting the correct answer.
    b. 40/60 chance of selecting the correct answer.
    c. 20/80 chance of selecting the correct answer.
    d. 50/50 chance of selecting the correct answer. ____

22. When writing a true/false test, do not use words such as:
    a. never.   **c.** always.
    b. usually.   **d.** all of the above. ____

23. When writing matching test questions, the educator should consider these guidelines:
    a. keep the sets to 25 items.
    b. items in the set should not be common to each other.
    c. the number of problems should exceed the matches.
    d. none of the above. ____

24. To eliminate subjectivity in scoring an essay test, the educator should:
    a. protect students' identity by assigning the students numbers that can be correlated to their names.
    b. first write a response to each question.
    c. review the response and make a notation on each important point.
    d. all of the above. ____

25. When constructing fill-in-the-blank questions:
    a. avoid writing styles that give the learners the answer.
    b. ensure that all questions begin and end on the same page of the test.
    c. keep the statements appropriate for the reading level of the learners.
    d. all of the above. ____

26. Completion, or fill-in-the-blank, questions are used to measure:
    a. recall learning.   c. prediction.
    b. higher-order thinking. d. none of the above. ____

27. In a multiple-choice question, the incorrect answers are known as:
    a. distracters or foils.   c. incorrect phrases.
    b. false answers.   d. impediments. ____

28. In a multiple-choice test, the difficulty of each question can be controlled by:
    a. the vagueness of the stem.
    b. how much alike the possible answers are.
    c. how much rambling there is in the question.
    d. the content of the subject. ____

29. To ensure consistency and objectivity when evaluating the practical skills of learners:
    a. educators will use evaluation scales to measure student performance on an individual basis.
    b. educators will use their mood to measure student performance on an individual basis.
    c. educators will use paper and pencil to measure student performance on an individual basis.
    d. none of the above. ____

30. A five-point rating scale ranging from "strongly agree" to "strongly disagree" or from "poor" to "excellent" is the simple:
    a. rating scale.   c. rubric.
    b. checklist.   d. Likert scale.   ____

31. A rating scale with fewer categories than the Likert scale that can be used to compare performance as well as work attitudes is the:
    a. rating scale.   c. rubric.
    b. checklist.   d. performance checklist.   ____

32. The rating scale known as the checklist would have categories such as:
    a. adequate/inadequate.   c. unsatisfactory.
    b. satisfactory.   d. all of the above.   ____

33. The type of evaluation that uses specific performance criteria in the rating process to ensure that a certain competency level has been reached is the:
    a. checklist.
    b. rubric.
    c. performance checklist.
    d. Likert scale.   ____

34. An advantage of using the performance checklist is that:
    a. it removes the opinion of the educator from the rating process.
    b. it is effective in preparing students for the state licensing examination.
    c. it is useful when determining if certain competency levels have been completed.
    d. all of the above.   ____

35. How is the performance checklist helpful to the educator?
    a. It gives the educator a quicker way to grade students, thereby reaching all students in a timely manner and leaving more time for paperwork.
    b. The educator has a hard copy to document each student's skill and chastise them on their work.
    c. The checklist is constructed in a way to minimize educator subjectivity and focus on whether or not the activity was performed as written.
    d. none of the above.   ____

36. The method of grading that incorporates scoring of more than one area of learner assessment is:
    a. point grading.
    b. multiple grading.
    c. multiple-category grading.
    d. all of the above. ____

37. In point grading, points are given to each criteria; this allows the educator to:
    a. ensure that the learner receives credit for performing the more difficult tasks correctly.
    b. place emphasis on the more important tasks to be completed during the evaluation.
    c. ensure that the learner receives credit for performing the more important tasks correctly.
    d. all of the above. ____

38. A clearly developed scoring document used to differentiate between levels of development in a specific activity and that may also be used as a self-assessment tool is the:
    a. rubric.   c. checklist.
    b. Likert scale.   d. rating scale. ____

39. A student whose academic or attendance progress is unsatisfactory must be advised and provided with:
    a. academic advisement and counseling.
    b. referral to professional assistance.
    c. any needed assistance.
    d. all of the above. ____

40. Educators may have the need to discuss the learner's work attitudes, professionalism, and compliance with the institution's code of conduct; the best place to do this is:
    a. in the lunchroom.
    b. when doing academic advisement counseling.
    c. in class.
    d. all of the above. ____

41. Student conferences should:
    a. have educator and student sit face to face.
    b. bring about change and not intimidate.
    c. be as nonthreatening as possible.
    d. all of the above. ____

42. During the conference the educator should practice:
    a. effective listening skills.
    b. monitoring of the student behavior.
    c. ignoring what the student is saying.
    d. the art of interjecting her own thoughts while the student is speaking. ____

43. A written agreement made between the learner and the educator determining agreed-upon behavior is a(n):
    a. promise.
    b. indemnity.
    c. guarantee.
    d. contract. ____

44. The purpose of a signed agreement is to:
    a. add meaning between the educator and learner.
    b. be signed by the educator and the leaner to document the commitment.
    c. instill a greater commitment to the agreed-upon behavior.
    d. all of the above. ____

45. Feedback on progress should be given to the learner:
    a. regularly.
    b. routinely.
    c. on a schedule.
    d. all of the above. ____

46. The essay form of testing may use higher-order thinking, but the responses become:
    a. subjective.
    b. objective.
    c. collective.
    d. none of the above. ____

47. When the educator unconsciously gives higher scores because of previous positive experience with a learner, this is:
    a. positive grading.
    b. personality grading.
    c. halo grading.
    d. radiant grading. ____

48. Grading a learner for higher-than-deserved achievement is:
    a. positive performance grading.
    b. grading improvement only.
    c. low/high performance.
    d. student reward grading. ____

49. Educators using "grading with warm fuzzies":
    a. want all learners to feel great.
    b. may lack confidence in their own skills.
    c. may lack understanding of grading procedures and criteria.
    d. all of the above. ____

50. Critical qualities of a master educator are:
    a. fairness and consistency.
    b. good grooming and good posture.
    c. decorum and stature.
    d. none of the above. ____

Part II
Supplementary Basic Teaching Skills for Career Education in Beauty and Wellness Disciplines

13 Making the Student Salon an Adventure

MULTIPLE CHOICE

1. Training received in the school clinic is vital to the success of the future graduate because:
   a. it makes real-world training experience part of their education.
   b. graduates make the transition from school to work more easily.
   c. students practice their people skills and sales techniques by working with the public.
   d. all of the above. ____

2. The students' success in the student salon will determine:
   a. entry-level success in the salon.
   b. successful habits.
   c. positive growth.
   d. all of the above. ____

3. Current research indicates that for optimum profit the school should attempt to generate clinic revenue that represents:
   a. 10 percent of the overall operating income.
   b. 15 percent of the overall operating income.
   c. 20 percent of the overall operating income.
   d. 25 percent of the overall operating income. ____

4. Researchers suggest that retail sales should generate:
   a. 5 percent of student salon revenue.
   b. 10 percent of student salon revenue.
   c. 15 percent of student salon revenue.
   d. 20 percent of student salon revenue. ____

5. Student tuition, including registration fees, books, and kits, constitutes:
   a. 75 percent of the overall revenue.
   b. 65 percent of the overall revenue.
   c. 55 percent of the overall revenue.
   d. 45 percent of the overall revenue. ____

6. Schools should expect a minimum net profit of 10 percent. If the net profit is greater than 10 percent, schools should consider sharing the profit with staff and faculty. If the school's annual financial statement results in less than a 10 percent profit:
   a. the school will show a decline and will soon be forced to close its doors and the staff will need to find other employment.
   b. all staff members and faculty must realize that there is a need to change. The operations should be evaluated and a plan of action implemented that will achieve the desired results.
   c. it is the responsibility of the owner to "fix" the situation and implement a plan of action.
   d. all of the above.   ____

7. Master educators will make the student salon a(n):
   a. adventure.   c. hazard.
   b. risky undertaking.   d. experience.   ____

8. To achieve important goals in life, science tells us that:
   a. emotion and hard work are highly effective.
   b. desire and compassion are highly effective.
   c. self-suggestion and visualization are highly effective.
   d. fortitude and hard work are highly effective.   ____

9. The ability to direct individual accomplishment toward the organization's objectives is:
   a. rivalry.   c. harmony.
   b. cooperation.   d. teamwork.   ____

10. For a team member to succeed:
    a. it is critical for each individual to understand their role and help the team member succeed.
    b. it takes a community of well-intentioned clients.
    c. it takes quality work, a winning smile, and talent.
    d. none of the above.   ____

11. For students to be highly successful, they need to understand that their personal role includes:
    a. how to hide from the instructor.
    b. gaining knowledge and building practical skills expertise.
    c. trying to get the client who tips well.
    d. none of the above.   ____

12. A successful student salon will see students:
    a. developing a positive, winning attitude and wearing a winning smile.
    b. developing a sound client base of at least 300 clients during a year.
    c. generating student salon revenue that ultimately contributes to the overall success of the school.
    d. all of the above. ____

13. _____support the student in the clinic salon.
    a. Salon clients
    b. Parents and other family of the student
    c. Educators and other staff members
    d. All of the above ____

14. Students who build a large clientele in the student salon are:
    a. able to gain maximum skill development.
    b. more likely to develop good sales techniques.
    c. gaining valuable experience necessary to make them highly competitive with seasoned professionals in the salon.
    d. all of the above. ____

15. Goals for a profitable student salon should be:
    a. worthwhile, predetermined, and realistic.
    b. made with high expectations, surreal, and predetermined.
    c. elusive, variable, and worthwhile.
    d. none of the above. ____

16. To provide an atmosphere that is inviting to the clients who enter the school:
    a. the owner should hire a good janitorial service and the team should criticize the janitorial work.
    b. the team should regularly survey the school from the front door to the back door to look for safety, cleanliness, and comfort.
    c. trust a student to check around the school and report back.
    d. all of the above. ____

17. Many times we forget that our students are the consuming public as well as the clients who take part in the clinic services. A disorderly and/or dirty reception area or student salon:
    a. will not make any difference in clients' perception of the school.
    b. will reflect badly on the image of the school and the education it provides.
    c. will give the impression to the students that the school is laid back and not led by drill sergeants.
    d. none of the above. ____

18. A good way for the team to get a true look at the school is to:
    a. take pictures and display them.
    b. hire a "secret shopper" to visit the school.
    c. periodically exit the front door and reenter as if entering the facility for the first time.
    d. get a copy of the state inspector's report. ____

19. The school receptionist position is important because:
    a. the receptionist not only schedules appointments, but also acts as a link between the client and the school.
    b. the reception area is the first thing clients and prospective student see when they arrive at school.
    c. the receptionist will never get a "second chance to make a positive first impression."
    d. all of the above. ____

20. The attitude of the receptionist is vital and should be:
    a. sugary sweet and flamboyant when answering the phone and dealing with the public.
    b. positive, smiling, and maintained at all times.
    c. pretentious and deceptive toward clients.
    d. grandiose, cheery, and maintained when greeting clients and answering the phone. ____

21. The reception area is the first thing clients and prospective students see when they arrive at the institution, so:
    a. master educators will ensure that every student is taught the important steps of managing a successful reception desk, from the telephone to the cash register.
    b. no one needs be involved in its operations.
    c. only the smartest students should be taught the important steps of managing a successful reception desk, from the telephone to the cash register.
    d. only students with disabilities should be taught the important steps of managing a successful reception desk, from the telephone to the cash register. ____

22. Because the reception area is the hub of the student salon, the master educator will ensure that the receptionist:
    a. thanks the clients as they leave; it's not important to offer rebooking.
    b. shows the client to a seat and then leaves the client there without assistance.
    c. offers retail or maintenance products to all clients.
    d. sets up the reception desk as the clients wait. ____

23. The public is now more aware of the importance of disease and infection control; thus, the master educator will:
    a. ensure that all students understand the importance of performing required infection control practices before and after each client visit.
    b. insist that students practice the highest degree of cleanliness throughout the day and leave stations shining at the end of the day.
    c. assign and monitor other general infection control duties that will ultimately leave the student salon in the best possible condition for the next day's services.
    d. all of the above. ____

24. The master educator will model throughout the day:
    a. infection control and cleaning.   c. teamwork.
    b. that no job is too small.   d. all of the above. ____

25. As a committed school team working toward the same goal:
    a. any untidiness will be taken care of, no matter who has been assigned that responsibility on that day.
    b. the facility and equipment will be monitored regularly.
    c. needed repairs will be reported to appropriate personnel in a timely manner.
    d. all of the above. ____

26. When students see that the master educator will do tasks needing to be done in school at random they:
    a. are grateful; now they do not have to perform their duties.
    b. think it is demeaning.
    c. think they are part of a working team and all are pulling together for a common goal.
    d. none of the above.

27. The master educator will ensure that each student understands the record-keeping responsibility of:
    a. a release form or hold harmless form that is signed by clients for all chemical services.
    b. certain client records that must be maintained by students.
    c. obtaining the client's signature on the release statement prior to the service.
    d. all of the above.

28. A release form or hold harmless form is required by some:
    a. school administrators.
    b. malpractice insurance companies.
    c. state boards.
    d. federal agencies.

29. The release form is used to:
    a. encourage clients to be truthful about prior chemical services.
    b. provide HIPPA regulations.
    c. obtain personal information.
    d. see the neighborhood of the client.

30. An important record is the client analysis and consultation form; the information that the master educator must ensure the student records is:
    a. analysis notes, predisposition test, strand test and whole-head results (applicable for chemical services), timing, and suggestions for the next service.
    b. analysis notes, timing, condition of scalp, product, cost, results, and suggestions for the next service.
    c. personal information, results, and suggestions for the next service.
    d. all of the above.

31. The dispensary attendant is responsible for:
    a. pulling the applicable client record form for each client.
    b. making sure no one comes into the dispensary.
    c. collecting student payment for all salon products used on the clients.
    d. selecting hair color. ____

32. Educators should make certain that dispensary attendants be taught:
    a. that it's too time-consuming to keep the dispensary clean.
    b. to stack new stock so the educator can inventory all of the new items.
    c. the importance of monitoring inventory control.
    d. to assign another student to perform distasteful tasks. ____

33. The most critical part of building a dynamic student salon is:
    a. how the clients are handled on the telephone.
    b. how the clients are handled from the moment they enter the school until the time they depart.
    c. how the clients are handled in the reception area.
    d. how the clients are handled when getting a shampoo. ____

34. The educator must instruct the students on the proper way to greet the client, as follows:
    a. "Good morning (afternoon, evening) Hon. How are you? I'm looking forward to giving you your color today. Come with me and we'll get started."
    b. "Good morning (afternoon, evening) Mrs. Banks. It sure has been cold out there today. I hope we get a break in the weather. Let's get started."
    c. "Hey, there. My name is Erin, how are you? Come with me and we'll get started."
    d. "Good morning (afternoon, evening) Mrs. Banks. My name is Erin, how are you? I'm looking forward to performing your color today. Please come with me and we'll get started." ____

35. It may be difficult to recognize first-time clients; thus the master educator will instruct the receptionist to:
    a. inform the student stylist.
    b. place a colored dot on the ticket.
    c. use a craft punch on the ticket.
    d. all of the above. ____

36. The master educator will be the model of good grooming; the following is true about students:
    a. students don't follow rules of good grooming.
    b. the way students dress and groom themselves is a reflection of their self-image and also reflects on the school and its clinic.
    c. if they wear a lab coat or smock no one will notice how the students are groomed.
    d. as long as the students come in to work in the student salon it doesn't matter if they are groomed for success. ____

37. The master educator will evaluate the appearance of the student daily using which of the following criteria?
    a. Is clothing clean, pressed, and free of stains and/or damage?
    b. Are shoes clean and polished?
    c. Are makeup and hair appropriate, nails well manicured, and jewelry and fragrance appropriate?
    d. All of the above. ____

38. Master educators will stress to the students that the clients they serve:
    a. are in for just a service.
    b. are just another ticket.
    c. are human beings and in need of pampering.
    d. are one more task closer to graduation. ____

39. Students should be taught to reflect after each client by asking:
    a. Did I greet the client warmly with a friendly smile and a handshake?
    b. Did the client leave a tip?
    c. Did the client compliment me on my work?
    d. Did the client tell the instructor how well I performed? ____

40. A tour of the facility will:
    a. be brief but also informative.
    b. familiarize clients with the surroundings so that they may be comfortable while there.
    c. familiarize clients with other students, especially those specializing in other disciplines.
    d. all of the above. ____

41. When students extend themselves, they are:
    a. interacting with clients by doing or saying a little bit more than necessary and making a lasting impression.
    b. doing the job of the educator.
    c. making money for the school and exerting more effort than necessary.
    d. faced with possible rejection from the client and hurt feelings. _____

42. The master educator will increase the confidence and experiences of the students and also increase the revenue of the institution by:
    a. teaching students how to rebook clients for future services.
    b. teaching students how to encourage repeat services.
    c. teaching students how to ask the client for referrals; clients who like what the student has done will likely tell someone else.
    d. all of the above. _____

43. When teaching students how to cultivate clientele, it is best in the beginning to:
    a. allow the students to pass out business cards to the clients without explanation; they should know what to do.
    b. allow the students to pass out business cards to the clients and give them clear direction (if not scripted), so that they will feel confident.
    c. allow the students to pass out business cards to the clients and give them clear direction, and be sure they pass them out every time a client comes into the student salon.
    d. none of the above. _____

44. Teaching students to upgrade tickets will benefit the client and:
    a. will develop a dynamic student salon.
    b. any add-on services will complement the hair, skin, or nails.
    c. if retail is purchased it will be specifically for a need of the client.
    d. all of the above. _____

45. Research shows that stylists only spend approximately:
    a. 30 percent of their time actually serving clients.
    b. 40 percent of their time actually serving clients.
    c. 50 percent of their time actually serving clients.
    d. 60 percent of their time actually serving clients. ____

46. Master educators know the importance of using downtime effectively; they have students:
    a. send appreciation cards to clients or call to remind clients of chemical appointments.
    b. take breaks.
    c. go to the lunch room and hang out.
    d. take some time to go to the mall or beauty supply store. ____

47. The student professional portfolio is a collection over time of the best work the student has accomplished during the training period; it:
    a. is a collection of before-and-after photographs of clients with the best hair, skin/makeup, and nails.
    b. is also effective in obtaining employment after graduation.
    c. all of the choices.
    d. can give the client a level of confidence in the student's ability to perform that special color or texture service that is being suggested. ____

48. Keeping students challenged to compete with themselves and with each other:
    a. creates enthusiasm.
    b. creates excitement.
    c. creates a sense of adventure.
    d. all of the above. ____

49. Zone teaching involves:
    a. one educator checking for safety, client protection and comfort, and teaching.
    b. one educator checking for release forms, client protection and safety, and teaching.
    c. one educator checking for safety, teaching, and escorting students and clients to the reception area.
    d. one educator checking for safety, client protection and comfort, and then conferring with other educators. ____

50. When master educators oversee the work of many students in the student salon:
   a. they use the clinic mirrors to observe several students at any one time.
   b. they must walk between students, assist them in completing a portion of the client's service, and then move on.
   c. they find one position and observe the entire clinic; when help is needed they can see and assist the student.
   d. there must be overhead mirrors installed to observe more than 15 students at one time. ____

51. Hair color services can prove to be problematic to the new student; thus the master educator will ensure that all students are properly trained in the formulation and application of hair color and:
   a. the removal of color from the client's skin.
   b. the removal of color from the floor.
   c. the removal of color from the chair back and arms.
   d. all of the above. ____

52. When performing demonstrations, the master educator:
   a. may leave the class for forgotten tools.
   b. may use the tools and equipment of a student.
   c. will plan ahead and have the necessary tools and supplies.
   d. will find it unnecessary to use infection control practices. ____

14 Career and Employment Preparation

MULTIPLE CHOICE

1. A summary of your education, work experience, achievements, and accomplishments is a:
   - **a.** resume.
   - **b.** cover letter.
   - **c.** job application.
   - **d.** portfolio. ____

2. When preparing your resume:
   - **a.** print it on good-quality bond paper and keep it to one page if possible.
   - **b.** include your name, address, phone number, and email address.
   - **c.** present recent, relevant work experience and relevant education.
   - **d.** all of the above. ____

3. Your resume should present concrete evidence of your skills and accomplishment, such as:
   - **a.** pictures of students at work with clients and in a theoretical class.
   - **b.** samples of student's work, such as nail art done on nail tips.
   - **c.** any special recognition or honors achieved while enrolled in a teacher training course.
   - **d.** lesson plans and accompanying handouts for a unit of instruction. ____

4. The employment portfolio is the vehicle you will use to show all your shining assets; although you may include a number of items, you should include:
   - **a.** diplomas, both secondary and postsecondary.
   - **b.** current resume focusing on accomplishments and including references.
   - **c.** professional affiliations, pictures of skills you have performed, and evaluations you have received.
   - **d.** all of the above. ____

5. Your portfolio should:
   a. be professionally prepared, typed, and tabbed for easy reference.
   b. be simple, with only four or five pages of accomplishments.
   c. include a history of your life accompanied with pictures from childhood.
   d. have attached references from close friends and relatives. ____

6. The document that explains why you chose to become an educator, your passion for the field, compassion for your students, and also describes methods or procedures you would employ to improve student outcomes and clinic and retail revenue is called a:
   a. personal mission statement.
   b. philosophy of teaching.
   c. dissertation of teaching.
   d. principle of teaching. ____

7. When pursuing a place of employment, you should consider:
   a. not waiting until after graduation to begin your search.
   b. the type of students and clients you wish to serve.
   c. each employer's advertisements for consistency, quality of ad, and what market they are targeting in the ad.
   d. all of the above. ____

8. An indirect method of job hunting that establishes contacts and allows you to distinguish between schools is:
   a. espionage.   c. networking.
   b. interconnect.   d. channeling. ____

9. If a school does not have an opening at the present time:
   a. ask them to retain your resume for later reference.
   b. thank them for their time.
   c. attend the interview anyway; it will give you experience.
   d. all of the above. ____

10. Appearance is important during an interview; you are applying for a position in an industry known to be on the cutting edge of style and beauty. Thus, you should:
    a. dress in the trendiest outfit; those in the position of hiring will think you are "in the know."
    b. choose an outfit that is comfortable, in perfect condition, and of a style and color that are flattering to your shape and personality.
    c. not worry too much about what you wear, just be sure your fragrance is bold and extreme.
    d. wear jewelry that reflects the current trend, show off your makeup talents, and flaunt your ability to use flamboyant accessories. ____

11. Being unprepared for an interview can be embarrassing; make sure to bring:
    a. your employment portfolio.
    b. your resume, even if one has been sent.
    c. facts and figures (employers, education, references, etc.).
    d. all of the above. ____

12. The entire interview can be made more comfortable if you reflect on possible questions that may be asked, such as:
    a. What is your ethnic background?
    b. How would you handle a problem student?
    c. What is your sexual preference?
    d. What is your religion? ____

13. During the employment interview:
    a. chew gum only if it is offered.
    b. project a serious image; no smiling.
    c. answer questions honestly.
    d. take your time to answer questions and show the interviewer your lecturing technique. ____

14. When interviewing, prepare questions for the employer ahead of time, such as:
    a. How much vacation time will I get?
    b. When will I receive my first raise?
    c. How soon will I be promoted?
    d. Is there room for advancement? ____

15. Congratulations! You have the job. To get to know your new place of employment:
    a. determine benefits package and payroll deductions.
    b. ascertain which regulatory agencies have oversight over the institution.
    c. obtain a copy of the school's operating procedures.
    d. all of the above. ____

16. Upon entering a new environment, the master educator will:
    a. attempt to change the school's curricula.
    b. rewrite all the currently used lesson plans.
    c. use a grading system different from the existing system.
    d. become familiar with the curricula and lesson plans, standards, grading, and other information. ____

17. If you find yourself a member of a school team that is rife with petty disagreements:
    a. quit.
    b. join the pettiness.
    c. keep a positive attitude.
    d. continue to be miserable. ____

18. When starting a new career, you should:
    a. avoid excess alcohol and tobacco and remain drug-free.
    b. exercise daily and wear well-fitting, comfortable shoes.
    c. get enough rest, drink plenty of water, and eat a balanced diet.
    d. all of the above. ____

19. Some basic factors to consider when undertaking the challenges of opening your own school include:
    a. the availability of a mall for students to visit.
    b. written agreements and a business plan.
    c. flyers to be printed.
    d. salons in the area. ____

20. When developing a business plan you will need to provide projected income and overhead expenses for up to:
    a. three years.   c. five years.
    b. four years.   d. six years. ____

21. Once you have hired a qualified consultant, chosen a good location, and complied with local and state licenses and regulations, you need:
    a. to know and comply with OSHA guidelines.
    b. insurance for malpractice, property liability, fire, burglary, theft, and business interruption.
    c. a system to record all financial activities that go on in the business as well as any other record keeping necessary.
    d. all of the above. ____

22. When the owner is the manager, decision maker, assumes the expenses, bears the losses, and receives the profits, the business is a:
    a. sole proprietorship.   c. corporation.
    b. partnership.   d. investment.   ____

23. When ownership is shared, although not necessarily equally, and partners also assume the other's unlimited liability for debts, the business is a(n):
    a. sole proprietorship.   c. corporation.
    b. partnership.   d. investment.   ____

24. Most people choose to incorporate:
    a. to save money on taxes.
    b. to limit personal financial liability.
    c. because it is easier to raise capital.
    d. all of the above.   ____

25. Skills required to run a people-oriented business include a knowledge of sound business principles and:
    a. pleasant personality, good leadership skills, and computer technology.
    b. aptitude, good judgment, and an understanding of fair practice.
    c. an excellent business sense, aptitude, good judgment, and diplomacy.
    d. an excellent business sense, good judgement, and an understanding of franchise opportunities.   ____

26. Business records are of value only if they are correct, concise, and complete. Which of the following statements concerning record keeping is correct?
    a. Income is usually classified as receipts from services and retail sales.
    b. Retain check stubs, canceled checks, receipts, and invoices.
    c. Expenses include rent, utilities, insurance, salaries, advertising, equipment, and repairs.
    d. All of the statements are correct. ____

27. Inventory and supplies need close monitoring to prevent:
    a. pilfering.
    b. damage.
    c. corrosion.
    d. instability. ____

28. For continued success in business and to have a thriving school, it is necessary to:
    a. offer refreshments to students and clinic clients.
    b. have incentive programs for students and clinic clients.
    c. remodel every two to four years to keep up with the trends.
    d. take remarkably good care of the students and clinic clients. ____

29. To ensure maximum efficiency when planning the layout of a school, you must consider:
    a. seeking the services of a reputable professional equipment supplier.
    b. acquiring the assistance of an architect.
    c. the programs you will offer and the number of students you will maintain, as well as the number of clients you will serve per day.
    d. all of the above. ____

30. Making good hiring decisions is critical; you must look for certain traits such as personal grooming, image as it relates to the school environment, overall attitude, and:
    a. communication skills and professionalism.
    b. communication skills and kindness.
    c. communication skills and creativity.
    d. communication skills and diligence. ____

31. For your team to feel appreciated for all their efforts you must be willing to share the success; whenever it is financially feasible to do so:
    a. offer hardworking and loyal employees as many benefits as possible.
    b. have an appreciation gathering each season.
    c. hold an award celebration whenever possible.
    d. a token gift at the holiday season is in order. ____

32. Managing others comes naturally to some but not to others; this skill:
    a. cannot be developed; you must be born with it.
    b. is possible to learn.
    c. is an intrapersonal gift.
    d. is an interpersonal gift. ____

33. The school receptionist is also the school's official greeter; other duties that may be included in the job description are:
    a. salesperson.
    b. answering the phone.
    c. taking appointment information.
    d. all of the above. ____

34. As the official greeter, the receptionist must possess an attractive appearance and:
    a. knowledge of the services offered at the school.
    b. knowledge of the programs offered and admission referral procedures.
    c. unlimited patience with both clients and school personnel.
    d. all of the above. ____

35. It is said that the person on the other end of the phone will hear the "smile" in your voice. When using the phone:
    a. you may have to speak loudly because of the clinic noise level.
    b. slang is acceptable if the client can understand what you are saying.
    c. clear your throat before speaking.
    d. be tactful and don't say anything to irritate the person on the other end of the line. ____

36. People will call the school to seek information about:
    a. setting up an appointment with the admissions representative.
    b. canceling or rescheduling appointments.
    c. the type of services offered at the school.
    d. all of the above. ____

37. When you do not have the information requested during a telephone conversation:
    a. offer to call the that person back with the information as soon as you have it.
    b. put the phone down and get the information.
    c. tell the person to call back.
    d. none of the above. ____

38. If your school's policy allows for appointments and the desired student practitioner is not available:
    a. suggest other times that the student practitioner is available.
    b. suggest another student practitioner.
    c. offer to call the client if an available opening should occur.
    d. all of the above. ____

39. When handling client complaints over the phone:
    a. tell the client that the responsible person is not in at the present time.
    b. respond with self-control, tact, and courtesy, no matter how trying the circumstances.
    c. tell the client that you do not have the correct information to help in this situation.
    d. hang up; you do not have to listen to a client who is upset and ill tempered. ____

40. An important element of a student's success in the industry is the knowledge of sales. Educators must take the opportunity to train students to:
    a. offer good advice to clients about services and products.
    b. make clients their top priority when it comes to giving them quality care, services, and products that they believe in.
    c. educate the client as to the positive aspects of the home care line of professional cosmetics.
    d. all of the above. ____

41. Master educators will take advantage of community speaking engagements to promote the school and the clinic by preparing well in advance and:
    a. speaking "off the cuff" to show professionalism.
    b. practicing extemporaneous speaking.
    c. realizing that without the proper preparation, the presentation could do more harm than good to the school.
    d. being confident that nothing will go wrong. ____

42. Being appreciative to the local community volunteers and other agencies by offering them all half-priced services is more effective than:
    a. planned advertising.
    b. speaking engagements.
    c. handing out flyers.
    d. all of the above. ____

43. Community service activities:
    a. provide more training for students.
    b. get students out of class.
    c. offer a day off for some educators.
    d. make the day shorter. ____

15 The Art of Retaining Students

MULTIPLE CHOICE

1. It is important that an institution be led by a set of agreed-upon and shared beliefs; in order to achieve this:
   a. each staff member must take ownership in the institution's philosophy.
   b. all staff members must write their own philosophy.
   c. all staff members must pay attention to themselves and not bother anyone.
   d. the owner of the institution must devise a way for external motivation. ____

2. Various regulatory oversight agencies that govern institutions mandate a level of accountability with respect to:
   a. clients who are attending the student salon.
   b. products that are used in the student salon.
   c. the rate of students who complete the program and find gainful employment.
   d. all of the above. ____

3. Institutions today will be known for their quality reputation and successful completion rate when:
   a. each member resists change.
   b. the entire system of the institution is quality based.
   c. the staff is divided between the evening staff and the day staff.
   d. all staff members have completed their master's degree. ____

4. Planning a successful student retention program is a necessity and the strategies planned should include:
   a. details.   c. modules.
   b. guides.   d. questions. ____

5. A statement that describes what the institution does, its purpose, what services the institution provides, and where it provides the services is referred to as a(n):
   a. mission statement.   c. value statement.
   b. objective.   d. vision statement. ____

6. An optimistic statement that outlines where the institution wants to be in the future is referred to as a(n):
   a. mission statement.
   c. value.
   b. objective.
   d. vision statement. ____

7. The responsibility of ensuring that everyone understands the vision of the institution rests with:
   a. anyone who volunteers.
   b. leadership.
   c. the receptionist.
   d. the student of the month. ____

8. When the institution's vision changes it will need to:
   a. allocate resources to facilitate the changes.
   b. establish an identity for itself.
   c. examine alternative courses of action.
   d. all of the above. ____

9. The assessment of the institution's performance against the stated mission and vision statement would best be made by:
   a. area salons that employ the institution's graduates.
   b. the students.
   c. the institution's graduates.
   d. all of the above. ____

10. Administrative personnel hired by the institution should have an understanding of an institution's operating procedures and:
    a. be familiar with all regulatory oversight requirements applicable to the institution.
    b. become familiar with the students, knowing each by name and socializing with them from time to time.
    c. be able to find the records the student requires at some later date.
    d. have a strong desire to reenter or begin beauty training in the near future. ____

11. The institution must operate in an ethical manner at all times; ways of manifesting this responsibility include:
    a. accounting policies.
    b. advertising policies.
    c. handling student issues.
    d. all of the above. ____

12. When an institution has a set of shared attitudes, values, goals, and practices, these are known as the institution's:

a. characteristics.　　　　c. values.

b. style.　　　　　　　　d. virtues.　　　____

13. As the institution takes on a personality of its own, all who walk through its doors:

a. should feel welcome.

b. will know it's a place to do business.

c. will have a professional-like service.

d. should know how to find their way out.　　　____

14. The institution's retention team consists of:

a. the owner, educators, and manager.

b. the owner, educator, manager, and receptionist.

c. the owner, educator, manager, and receptionist.

d. everyone, from the owners to the janitorial staff.　　　____

15. People can be trained in skills, but it is much more difficult to train them:

a. in computer technology.

b. in sales techniques.

c. to have a positive attitude.

d. in the use of audiovisual equipment.　　　____

16. When adults enroll in an institution, it is not to be expected that school is their only priority; at the admissions interview it would be prudent to make the student aware of:

a. policies and procedures.

b. complete costs involved in completion and certification and licensure.

c. course syllabi and grading.

d. all of the above.　　　____

17. A thorough orientation program is essential for student retention to:

a. promote a quality student salon.

b. prevent withdrawal later.

c. get to meet new students.

d. introduce the staff.　　　____

18. As the student comes to buy into the ownership of the institution, the institution's reputation in the community will grow and:
   a. there will be more clients and students.
   b. bills will keep getting larger.
   c. clients will have to wait.
   d. students will want more educators.   ____

19. Giving the adult learner some involvement in the policy-making and decision-making processes will:
   a. cause a catastrophe.
   b. set unrealistic policies.
   c. provide ownership of these processes.
   d. set absurd policy; they know nothing about running a learning center.   ____

20. Periodic feedback from students should be encouraged and valued; some insight for this strategy would be:
   a. students must sign the suggestion.
   b. all suggestions must be responded to.
   c. suggestions not acted upon must be responded to.
   d. all of the above.   ____

21. Many people say that curriculum is primarily two parts:
   a. content and delivery.
   b. cognitive and affective.
   c. theoretical and practical.
   d. verbal and nonverbal.   ____

22. The most important ingredient of a successful retention plan is the:
   a. students in class.
   b. energetic and effective educators.
   c. layout of the institution.
   d. student lounge.   ____

23. Institutions must take extreme care in considering the educational model they want to adopt; the model should focus on:
    a. promoting the skills of the students by having them in the student salon, to the detriment of their theoretical studies.
    b. educating the students on the products in the showcase, so that students can force them on the clients.
    c. promoting the other programs that the institution has to offer and guiding the students into taking more training.
    d. development of skills and abilities appropriate to the career the students have chosen. ____

24. Important qualities to develop in the classroom are:
    a. fidelity and compassion.
    b. excitement and love of learning.
    c. tenacity and a love of learning.
    d. self-esteem and compassion. ____

25. For education to be gratifying for the students, the educator will need to identify:
    a. their learning styles.
    b. their mood swings.
    c. if they are "morning" or "afternoon" people.
    d. their food preferences. ____

26. Effective teaching and classroom management are important to the organization of a classroom; as educators you will also develop methods to:
    a. teach students how to study.
    b. teach students how to take tests.
    c. excite every learner.
    d. all of the above. ____

27. As a master educator it is important that you make education exciting; therefore:
    a. show two-hour-long comedies about salons in class.
    b. take an hour or more and have students tell their favorite jokes.
    c. interject some humor in every lesson.
    d. have students download sites from the Internet that are funny. ____

28. The adult generally comes into the institution with a serious reason for training and may also have outside responsibilities; when dealing with the adult population:
   a. avoid taking the traditional teacher approach, meant for much younger people, with them.
   b. see students as clients and respect them.
   c. offer them choices but remind them of accreditation and regulatory guidelines that define what we can and cannot do.
   d. all of the above. ____

29. Faced with students of various diversities, we might _____ to determine how a strategy might affect a particular student.
   a. consult the Internet
   b. check with the university
   c. ask the admissions director
   d. simply ask the student ____

30. Providing customer service for learners does not have to be time consuming if we:
   a. are available for the learners to communicate to them our concern and willingness to support their goals.
   b. provide additional resources available for them when asked.
   c. address our comments to the individual student's goals.
   d. all of the above. ____

31. Students really don't care about our problems; they are interested in how we care about them. Some strategies to assist us are:
   a. it's not necessary to show appreciation to the students.
   b. listen to the student; it shows that you understand their needs.
   c. talk only to one or two students with whom you trust.
   d. try not to anticipate their needs; it gets frustrating to have a know-it-all around. ____

32. All teachers are in need of professional development; the ultimate responsibility lies with the:
   a. educator.   **c.** regulatory agency.
   b. manager.   **d.** owner.   ____

33. To ensure each educator receives professional development, each institution should have:
    a. a plan for all educators requiring them to meet their state requirements for license renewal.
    b. a plan for all educators to renew their accrediting agency requirements for professional development.
    c. written professional development plans for continuing education for all instructors in the institution.
    d. all of the above. ____

34. Methods of providing motivation include:
    a. keeping the institution in pristine condition.
    b. allowing instructor participation in the design of the institution's vision.
    c. allowing instructor participation in the design of the institution's culture.
    d. all of the above. ____

35. The desire for a stable work environment with equal opportunity for learning and personal growth is what educators ask for; the organization, in return:
    a. should be provided the same concern, respect, and caring attitude.
    b. expects hard work and dedication.
    c. expects educators to do their job of providing education to the students.
    d. should be provided respect, loyalty, and undying gratitude. ____

36. Educators who want to be on the cutting edge of education will:
    a. look at fashion magazines.
    b. watch the STYLE channel.
    c. attend seminars and conventions.
    d. all of the above. ____

37. The single most important action an educator can take to prevent a withdrawal is to:
    a. criticize.   c. praise.
    b. respect.   d. appreciate. ____

38. Performance will be improved if the educator praises the student:
    a. five times for every criticism.
    b. six times for every criticism.
    c. seven times for every criticism.
    d. eight times for every criticism. ____

39. Research has found that teachers praise only one time for every four criticisms; strategies for praise that may be considered include:
    a. praise can wait; it does not have to be immediate.
    b. general praise is as good as individual praise.
    c. sharing with the student how the performance made you feel as an educator.
    d. identifying the specific reasons you are offering praise. ____

40. Research shows that 15 to 20 percent of the institution's faculty will be the top performers and:
    a. everyone else in the middle are positive.
    b. 15 to 20 percent fall at the other end of the scale.
    c. the ones in the middle are passively positive.
    d. the ones in the middle are at the other end of the scale. ____

41. Most of the attention should be placed on the educators:
    a. at the bottom; they need the most help.
    b. in the middle, the bulk of need.
    c. at the top; these people will bring the others up to a higher expectation.
    d. all of the above. ____

42. Trust is an essential piece of the recognition process; it must mean the same for:
    a. administrators and students.
    b. support staff and clients.
    c. teachers and management.
    d. students and clients. ____

43. Institution staff, like your students, enjoy individual recognition; a vehicle for providing an uplifting morale booster would be a:
    a. small gift of appreciation.
    b. certificate of recognition.
    c. nonmonetary token of appreciation.
    d. all of the above. ____

44. For praise to be of value to the student it must be:
    a. sincere.   c. effective.
    b. spontaneous.   d. all of the above. ____

45. In our culture, using one's name while looking them in the eye conveys:

    a. aggression.   **c.** reverence.

    b. respect.   **d.** superiority.   ____

46. The more the student acts in a praiseworthy way:

    a. the more criticism is necessary.

    b. the less criticism is necessary.

    c. the sooner the praise can stop.

    d. the sooner an educator's job is done.   ____

47. When evaluating student performance:

    a. a systematic method of evaluation should be used throughout the program.

    b. a subjective method of evaluation should be used throughout the program.

    c. educators should develop their own evaluation systems to be used throughout the program.

    d. try different methods of evaluation; it is not necessary to be systematic.   ____

48. In order to improve performance the educator should:

    a. take frequent breaks.

    b. review material just before class.

    c. perform self-evaluations.

    d. prevent fatigue.   ____

49. As educators we cannot excite our students if:

    a. our pay scale does not meet our needs at the time.

    b. we are having a bad day.

    c. we do not have passion for the field we teach.

    d. the environment is not to our liking.   ____

50. Institution employees must be:

    a. light-hearted, dedicated, and skilled in the field.

    b. fully trained, qualified, and experienced to achieve the institution's mission and vision as well as educational objectives.

    c. dedicated to the task of training students to pass qualifying licensing exams and appropriate standards.

    d. skilled in the field.   ____

Part III

Professional Development for Career Education Instructors

16 Educator Relationships

MULTIPLE CHOICE

1. A connection or association that people have or a mutual dealing or working arrangement with others is referred to as a:
   a. similarity.
   b. relationship.
   c. rapport.
   d. marriage. ____

2. A master educator will develop a relationship with:
   a. learners and their family members.
   b. administrative personnel.
   c. other faculty members.
   d. all of the above. ____

3. Someone with whom you only communicate occasionally, and don't have a relationship with, is known as a mere:
   a. acquaintance.
   b. chance meeting.
   c. friend.
   d. associate. ____

4. For a relationship to last over time:
   a. it takes very little effort on the part of each of the individuals.
   b. one person must always give in to the request of the other.
   c. it must be continuous, perpetuated, and requires mutuality.
   d. there is relatively no risk involved. ____

5. It is said that good relationships are built on:
   a. scorn and tolerance.
   b. repudiation and understanding.
   c. mutual communication and require mutual investment.
   d. understanding and disdain. ____

6. Because you want to be able to satisfy the needs of people but you cannot always do so, this leads to:
   a. misunderstanding.
   b. tension.
   c. emotional stress.
   d. all of the above. ____

7. When our personal security is threatened we might not behave well and may react in a way that is:
   a. uncooperative, hostile, or withdrawn.
   b. angry and suspicious.
   c. worried, anxious, and overwhelmed.
   d. all of the above. ____

8. When feeling secure in our environment and our interaction with people, we will:
   a. refuse to give an opinion.
   b. be reluctant to take help from others.
   c. take pride in our ability to help others.
   d. refuse to interact with others. ____

9. Rude and insensitive people will be with us periodically; try to remember:
   a. that at this particular time these people feel insecure.
   b. not to let these people get away with it!
   c. to give them "an eye for an eye."
   d. to put them in their place. ____

10. Handling difficult situations can be distressing and drain your energy; thus:
    a. talk more and listen less.
    b. trust in other people's judgement.
    c. never agree with an angry client.
    d. respond and instead of reacting. ____

11. When you approach a new student:
    a. smile and be polite.   c. be inviting.
    b. be genuinely friendly.   d. all of the above. ____

12. Communication is a skill that can be expressed through many tools; as a master educator you will:
    a. use magnetic boards.
    b. cultivate effective listening skills.
    c. use graphs when necessary.
    d. use all electronic devices when necessary. ____

13. When speaking to clients or students, listening to the *whole person* means:
    a. being eager to hear what the speaker has to say.
    b. removing any other person in the area.
    c. gaining insight on the speaker's home life situation.
    d. considering the speaker's temperament, attitude, emotions, intellect, and speaking ability. ____

14. When we practice effective listening we find that it will:
    a. solve problems by allowing the speaker and listener to clarify their own thinking about the topic.
    b. decrease job performance by taking too much time.
    c. tune out our own opinions and ideas and focus only on the speaker's.
    d. distance ourselves from the problem and focus on another task. ____

15. Showing genuine interest in all those you teach can be accomplished with a:

    a. short survey of their interests.

    b. five-minute meeting with four or five students each day.

    c. lunchtime meeting with one or two students each day.

    d. conference after school.   ____

16. When having a meeting with the student:

    a. make one specific observation about the student.

    b. ask if there are any questions or concerns that the student would like to share.

    c. ask if the student has any needs.

    d. all of the above.   ____

17. To develop a true relationship with the learner:

    a. remove any negative expressions from your demeanor and be cheerful.

    b. know the name of each learner and pronounce it correctly.

    c. steer the learner toward ideas and conclusions don't do all the talking.

    d. all of the above.   ____

18. Master educators will search for ways to meet the needs of the learner; those needs may include:

    a. the need for acceptance as an individual.

    b. the need to overcompensate for lack of abilities.

    c. the need to strengthen inadequacies.

    d. all of the above.   ____

19. The master educator will make learners feel important when they:

    a. project a positive image.

    b. answer questions correctly.

    c. demonstrate quality practical work.

    d. all of the above.   ____

20. All institutions have standards and rules to ensure order in the classroom; however, when a student has made an unwise choice about a past infraction:

    a. remind the student about the failure to follow rules at each opportunity.

    b. make the student feel guilty about the past misdeed.

    c. the student should not be made to feel guilty about the unpleasant action.

    d. all of the above.   ____

21. Some educators will add a criticism to the praise they offer a student, sending a mixed message. Master educators will concentrate their energies on the development of:
    a. student's clear understanding of the message.
    b. student self-esteem.
    c. student self-confidence and self-respect.
    d. all of the above. ____

22. When a reprimand seems to be in order, remember to:
    a. formulate your rebuttals before the student has finished speaking.
    b. jump to conclusions before listening to the student responses to save time.
    c. use clarification and caring before confrontation if problems are to be solved.
    d. approach the problem with sternness. ____

23. Correcting a learner's performance can be difficult. Of importance is to:
    a. make your instructions clear, concise, and easy to follow.
    b. give lots of descriptors and negatives.
    c. be highly descriptive about the performance, using the word *but* frequently.
    d. ignore correct learner performances. ____

24. Some educators will gratify their own egos by making students feel inferior, such as by:
    a. focusing attention on all learners.
    b. appropriate use of praise.
    c. promoting self-esteem.
    d. generating student guilt. ____

25. When educators give too much praise to the learner:
    a. it can be a detriment.
    b. students may see it as insulting.
    c. the educator may seem insincere.
    d. all of the above. ____

26. The master educator will make it possible for every student to express personal feelings by ensuring that:
    a. respectful attention is given to the brightest students.
    b. unrealistic statements are ridiculed.
    c. questions that do not pertain to the subject matter must not be asked.
    d. respectful attention is given to an honest expression of the students' attitudes, ideas, concerns, and doubts. ____

27. Competition in the classroom should be encouraged:
   a. within students rather than with others.
   b. because it stimulates learning in every learner.
   c. because it discourages high achievers.
   d. to put everyone on an equal playing field. ____

28. One of the most important relationships an educator must develop is relationships with:
   a. guest speakers.   **c.** clients.
   b. other educators.   **d.** sales representatives. ____

29. Teamwork is the ability for educators to work together toward a common vision. If you choose not to be a member of the school team:
   a. you cannot be a loner and be appreciated or accepted by everyone else.
   b. other educators cannot relate to you if you purposely set yourself apart.
   c. you will not get much respect; educators will generally feel more respect for educators who are inclusive rather than exclusive.
   d. all of the above. ____

30. When other educators experience success:
   a. share in the joy.
   b. acknowledge the success immediately.
   c. become an advocate of the achievement.
   d. all of the above. ____

31. When a plan or idea must be conveyed to another individual or the group who will be working with the idea, it is referred to as:
   a. the transfer technique.   **c.** entitlement.
   b. transmission of ownership.   **d.** displaced ownership. ____

32. Criticizing the work of other educators will:
   a. damage the school's reputation.
   b. damage your relationship with others.
   c. ultimately reflect on you.
   d. all of the above. ____

33. Speaking "off the record":
   a. is not a good practice; many staff conflicts have occurred over this practice.
   b. is highly encouraged because it facilitates communication.
   c. ensures facts will be shared among team members.
   d. is a skill that must be practiced. ____

34. If you are missing information:
   a. say, "Nobody tells me anything."
   b. grumble and mutter expletives.
   c. request more staff meetings and an agenda.
   d. none of the above.   ____

35. When angry, you should handle the situation by:
   a. walking away and leaving the premises.
   b. speaking calmly and clarifying your position, being specific, and revealing a sense of responsibility.
   c. clamming up and leaving things alone; no one will listen to you anyway.
   d. counting to 10 to think it through; walking out if you are still upset.   ____

36. Master educators are eager to share information because:
   a. when helping other educators they also become successful.
   b. they always return information that has been lent.
   c. it benefits everyone if information, materials, and equipment are not hoarded.
   d. all of the above.   ____

37. Learning to handle criticism with a professional attitude will be beneficial to you; thus:
   a. don't whine, cry, or blame others.
   b. be honest and open; admit mistakes.
   c. be humble; criticism won't hurt as much.
   d. all of the above.   ____

38. Gossip should not be engaged in by educators because:
   a. speaking negatively about a colleague will make you appear untrustworthy.
   b. those listening will fear that you will speak the same way toward them.
   c. you must set high standards for students and yourself.
   d. all of the above.   ____

39. When introducing change in your institution:
   a. be forceful and leave tact behind.
   b. there may be roadblocks ahead of you, but you must knock them over; remember your ideas are best.
   c. know that the benefits must outweigh the personal prejudices other educators may hold.
   d. all of the above.   ____

40. It is difficult to be open-minded and see the "big picture" when:
   a. we look for the disadvantages rather than the advantages of a new concept.
   b. we are overly critical of new ideas and change.
   c. we are not supportive of new ideas and are not proactive to change.
   d. all of the above.   ____

41. The educator who is willing to stay abreast of current trends within the field of education:
   a. feels that "our school is different."
   b. faces challenges head-on with the intention of resolving them.
   c. is reluctant to experiment.
   d. will not look to the future for ways to improve.   ____

42. Exercising your right to know and keeping others informed will:
   a. cause staff friction; only key personnel need to know valuable information.
   b. remind key people within your institution that they are important to you and that you rely on them as a source of relevant and valuable information.
   c. make some staff feel superior and that they are very important.
   d. turn an ally into a foe.   ____

43. Master educators will respond professionally to unplanned situations by:
   a. developing a control mechanism.
   b. pouting for a planned amount of time.
   c. developing a tolerance for frustration.
   d. sulking until the situation changes.   ____

44. In order to form a powerful network with other master educators:
   a. the educator will identify problems constantly.
   b. the educator will present problems to colleagues.
   c. the educator will assume the responsibility of offering three solutions to every problem.
   d. all of the above.   ____

45. Regarding the curriculum offered in the institution you are working, it is to be respected and followed diligently; however:

    a. follow procedures to implement any needed improvements.

    b. change the curriculum as you see fit.

    c. implement the improvements without the approval of the institution.

    d. all of the above. _____

46. To ensure positive professional relationship with one's superiors:

    a. present problems to be solved.

    b. follow the educator position description and duties of the job.

    c. make superiors aware of others' errors.

    d. exercise initiative, starting work but not necessarily finishing. _____

47. Those in supervisory capacity will find it positive when educators:

    a. pay close attention to instructions and essential details.

    b. provide thorough and accurate reports when required.

    c. develop and convey self-confidence at all times.

    d. all of the above. _____

48. The rights of parents regarding their children's educational records:

    a. transfer to the student who has reached the age of 18.

    b. are governed by FERPA.

    c. transfer to the student who is attending any school beyond the high school level.

    d. all of the above. _____

49. The law allows schools to disclose records without consent to:

    a. appropriate parties in connection with financial aid to a student.

    b. parents when a student, who is over age 18, is still dependent.

    c. accrediting organizations.

    d. all of the above. _____

50. Master educators should be ambassadors of goodwill for the institutions they represent. By influencing the public's attitude toward the cosmetology school, educators are sharing:
   a. the lessons being taught.
   b. the various services and products that are offered by the school.
   c. the type of teaching strategies used.
   d. the type of procedures taught. ____

51. Public relations can be approached from many angles. By providing services to the community:
   a. you have established a positive, professional relationship that will serve students and the institution.
   b. you will deplete your inventory.
   c. you will have difficulty rebuilding your regular clientele; there will not be enough students to go around.
   d. all of the above. ____

CHAPTER **17** **Learning Is a Laughing Matter**

MULTIPLE CHOICE

1. Research tells us that the best conditions for learning are those that allow the student to feel safe enough to take risks. Some of the risks include:
   a. raising of the hand for some students.
   b. getting it wrong.
   c. peer disapproval.
   d. all of the above. ____

2. When educators create a sense of security for students it allows for:
   a. shared positive experiences.
   b. an indifferent attitude from students.
   c. student anxiety.
   d. underachievement and lack of creativity. ____

3. Sharing laughter in the classroom makes everyone feel safer and more comfortable; laughter produces:
   a. antihistamines.   c. interferons.
   b. dopamines.   d. endorphins. ____

4. Using humor in the classroom will make the students feel:
   a. that the educator is a buffoon.
   b. more responsive to learning.
   c. that the educator does not know the subject matter.
   d. uncomfortable. ____

5. The more positive and enduring the relationship you have with a class, the more risks you can take with humor; however:
   a. what you find humorous, students may not.
   b. when in doubt, toss it out.
   c. be cautious about exposing yourself to "ribbing."
   d. all of the above. ____

6. When a smile is genuine the muscle that is affected is the:
   a. zygomatic.   b. risorius.
   c. caninus.   d. mentalis. ____

7. Studies have proven that laughter and humor can be helpful in delivering curriculum content:
   a. by having the students laugh out loud.
   b. by having the students tell a funny story.
   c. by holding the attention of the learner.
   d. by getting the students to tell funny jokes. ____

8. Many positive effects are achieved by providing humor in the classroom, such as:
   a. being helpful in delivering curriculum.
   b. gaining the attention of the learner.
   c. aiding the retention of the information.
   d. all of the above. ____

9. The formal name given for the physiological study of humor and laughter and their effects on the human body is:
   a. gelotology.   c. myology.
   b. osteology.   d. gerontology. ____

10. Many believe that the purpose of laughter is to:
    a. produce negative emotions.
    b. hold in stress.
    c. strengthen human relationships.
    d. fill the body with unhealthy chemistry. ____

11. Laughter occurring when the outcome is different from what is expected is explained by:
    a. superiority theory.   c. relief theory.
    b. incongruity theory.   d. spontaneity theory. ____

12. When laughter occurs after a long period of tension, stress, suspension, or danger it is explained by the:
    a. superiority theory.   b. incongruity theory.
    c. relief theory.   d. spontaneity theory. ____

13. Laughter will open us up for maximum learning opportunities because it:
    a. increases stress.
    b. promotes anxiety.
    c. provides humiliation.
    d. improves our mental well-being. ____

14. The benefits of laughter include:
    a. more positive and optimistic mood.
    b. greater sense of control.
    c. emotional release.
    d. all of the above. _____

15. Many times we store negative emotions such as sadness, fear, and anger. Laughter can actually provide a harmless release of these emotions because laughter is:
    a. a detriment.   c. problematic.
    b. cathartic.   d. futile. _____

16. Regardless of language, age, or cultural background, laughter is considered:
    a. timeless.
    b. cleansing.
    c. the universal language.
    d. satisfying. _____

17. When there is laughter in the workplace there is:
    a. better conflict management.   c. more competition.
    b. more jealousy.   d. backbiting. _____

18. When you laugh with colleagues:
    a. communication skills improve.
    b. team building improves.
    c. there is greater morale.
    d. all of the above. _____

19. A characteristic of good humor on the job is that:
    a. creativity will be enhanced.
    b. stress will be increased.
    c. productivity will decrease.
    d. health will suffer. _____

20. Being able to bounce back and learn to adapt to the funnier side of everyday situations shows that you are:
    a. inflexible.   c. rigid.
    b. resilient.   d. unadaptable. _____

21. The feelings of optimism and well-being we receive from laughter are attributed to the production of:
    a. antihistamines.   c. endorphins.
    b. spondylitis.   d. gelotology. _____

22. It is known that laughter can improve physical health because it:
    a. provides an excellent source of cardiac exercise.
    b. reduces carbon monoxide in the lungs.
    c. increases water vapor in the lungs.
    d. increases infectious organisms entering the respiratory tract. ____

23. The physical health benefits of laughter include:
    a. clearing the respiratory tract.
    b. strengthens the immune system.
    c. reduces stress hormones.
    d. all of the above. ____

24. One of the physical health benefits of laughter is weight loss. Research indicates:
    a. 100 hearty laughs will burn the same amount of calories as a 10-minute jog.
    b. 100 hearty laughs will burn the same amount of calories as a triathlon.
    c. 100 hearty laughs will burn the same amount of calories as a three-mile run.
    d. all of the above. ____

25. It has been said that:
    a. 30 seconds of laughter is worth 30 minutes of deep relaxation.
    b. 1 minute of laughter is worth 40 minutes of deep relaxation.
    c. 90 seconds of laughter is worth 50 minutes of deep relaxation.
    d. 2 minutes of laughter is worth 60 minutes of deep relaxation. ____

26. The most rampant disease in our country today is said to be:
    a. burnout.   c. Epstein-Barr.
    b. stress.   d. hernia. ____

27. When the educator knows how to effectively interject humor into the content of the lesson and strives to seek ways to improve its use, this is referred to as:
    a. conscious incompetence.
    b. conscious competence.
    c. unconscious incompetence.
    d. unconscious competence. ____

28. When the educator has a deficit in the humor department and neither understands humor in education nor has a desire to address it, this may be referred to as:
a. unconscious incompetence.
b. conscious incompetence.
c. unconscious competence.
d. conscious competence. ____

29. When the master educator's humor is spontaneous, warm, and appropriate, it's "second nature," it can be referred to as:
a. unconscious incompetence.
b. conscious incompetence.
c. conscious competence.
d. unconscious competence. ____

30. In humans the part of the brain involved in motivation and emotional behaviors is the:
a. thalamus gland.   c. hippocampus.
b. limbic system.   d. amygdala. ____

31. As educators, the type of humor we would like to establish in the classroom is:
a. unconscious incompetence.
b. conscious incompetence.
c. conscious competence.
d. unconscious competence. ____

32. As educators, we have the ability to instill:
a. self-esteem.   c. self-acceptance.
b. love of learning.   d. all of the above. ____

33. Self-talk is an internal dialogue that can influence our emotional state. The master educator can teach students that positive self-talk must always be performed in the personal tense and:
a. the present tense.
b. with enthusiasm.
c. with visualization of the praise and accolades.
d. all of the above. ____

34. How do ideas arise? When does creativity take place?
a. by talking with others
b. by brainstorming
c. through transfer of ideas
d. all of the above ____

35. Students who feel that they are not creative or are troubled
    about lack of talent should be reminded that:
    a. creativity is within all of us.
    b. we can self-talk our way to creativity.
    c. if we believe it we can achieve it.
    d. all of the above.   ____

36. Rejection of an idea is difficult, but to a student it can be
    cutting. We need to impress on the learner that the next
    idea will be better and have the student:
    a. repeat that technique or idea.
    b. sulk in the lunch area.
    c. combine that technique with another.
    d. none of the above.   ____

37. If we find that we are at a stalemate during a creative
    process, the best thing to do is:
    a. walk away for 20 minutes then finish the work.
    b. stand up, walk away, and spend five minutes
       daydreaming.
    c. stand, walk away, daydream for five minutes, and get
       right back to work.
    d. walk away for 10 minutes and then finish the work.   ____

38. We need to help students become people of "action."
    Learners must follow through with a good idea, so
    encourage them to:
    a. write an action plan.
    b. establish a deadline.
    c. list the required necessary tasks.
    d. all of the above.   ____

39. Humor in the workplace provides an atmosphere of:
    a. team spirit.   c. fun.
    b. goodwill.   d. all of the above.   ____

40. As master educators we can create a fun work environment
    in such ways as:
    a. spending five minutes laughing on the way to work.
    b. reading the newspaper.
    c. working on lesson plans.
    d. doing our taxes.   ____

41. It is hard to be angry with someone you have had fun with earlier, such as:
    a. having snacks within the teacher's room.
    b. in a huddle before the day begins.
    c. sharing birthday cake with.
    d. all of the above.   ____

42. Master educators must come to class prepared for anything, so it is prudent to be prepared with a type of kit made expressly for the humor classroom referred to as the:
    a. first aid kit.   c. glee aid kit.
    b. mirth aid kit.   d. laugh aid kit.   ____

43. When there is a lull in the class, you might allow the students to participate in reading a collection of preapproved:
    a. stories or G-rated jokes.
    b. trade journal articles.
    c. fashion magazines.
    d. local newspaper articles.   ____

44. Use of inspirational stories and video clips serves a purpose during the course of training. Use them to create:
    a. a feeling of warmth.   b. a feeling of safety.
    c. a feeling of comfort.   d. all of the above.   ____

45. The older we grow the less we laugh; children laugh about 400 times per day while adults laugh:
    a. 5 times per day.   b. 20 times per day.
    c. 15 times per day.   d. 20 times per day.   ____

46. Giving projects funny names or incorporating the elements of a game into the class:
    a. serves no purpose.
    b. makes the time go faster but the learning go slower.
    c. wastes valuable time.
    d. none of the above.   ____

18 Teaching Success Strategies for a Winning Career

MULTIPLE CHOICE

1. A student's _____ and _____ developed in school will determine the type of career they will have later.
   a. prosperity, spending
   b. goal-setting, saving
   c. mediocrity, lack of skill
   d. activities, habits _____

2. The principles that master educators want their students to follow include value yourself, motivate yourself, expect to win, manage your goals, and
   a. adopt a strong work ethic.   c. focus on fun.
   b. market your potential.   d. polish your potential. _____

3. Highly successful people have a strong inner feeling of their own:
   a. flaws.   c. assets.
   b. worth and value.   d. detriments. _____

4. Believing in yourself allows you to use all your potential to take action and achieve results. This positive behavior is known as:
   a. managing yourself.   c. valuing yourself.
   b. managing your goals.   d. expecting to win. _____

5. In order to build a strong self-belief and sense of self-esteem, have students:
   a. identify what they view as their core values.
   b. ask a friend to select their core values.
   c. ask their parents what their core values should be.
   d. adopt the values of a friend. _____

6. You practice your self-worth when you:
   a. sit in the last row.
   b. look your best and walk tall.
   c. slouch.
   d. keep to yourself and speak to no one. _____

7. Everyone loves the sound of their name; teach learners to pay value to their names by:
   a. introducing themselves first by name.
   b. using their names in conversation.
   c. stating their names at the beginning of every phone call.
   d. all of the above.   ____

8. When we take time to develop a plan for self-improvement and individualized development, we might refer to it as:
   a. finding our learning style.
   b. planning our activities.
   c. planning our growth.
   d. developing career education.   ____

9. When someone pays a compliment to another it is courteous to say "thank you"; if you negate the compliment:
   a. you disrespect yourself.
   b. the person may consider you rude.
   c. it suggests to the person paying the compliment that it was meaningless.
   d. all of the above.   ____

10. As educators we have high expectations for our students; we must also foster an attitude of positive expectancy and:
    a. develop an attitude of inadequacy.
    b. develop an attitude of abandon.
    c. create a definite purpose for life.
    d. cultivate disregard.   ____

11. Master educators know that external motivators will only last a short time; it is our responsibility to help the learner understand that:
    a. true motivation is internal.
    b. self-motivation is critical for success.
    c. the energy for self-motivation lies in the learner's visions for the future.
    d. all of the above.   ____

12. When learners are internally motivated they will be in control and:
    a. be less likely to take up new activities.
    b. take unrealistic chances.
    c. be discouraged by setbacks.
    d. maintain enthusiasm about life.   ____

13. If the learner is motivated by desire and not by fear, the outcome will be:
    a. destructive.
    c. successful.
    b. negative.
    d. annihilative.   ____

14. Because, as the saying goes, "You can't soar like an eagle, when you work with turkeys," we must teach the learner to:
    a. move toward negative influences.
    b. move toward positive concepts.
    c. take flying lessons.
    d. ignore negative people.   ____

15. When self-motivation wanes, try:
    a. to do something you love doing.
    b. beating yourself up emotionally.
    c. thinking of all the failures you have had in the past.
    d. calling a friend who likes to complain.   ____

16. Ways to renew your self-motivation include:
    a. changing your vocabulary.
    b. listing your desires.
    c. reviewing your successes.
    d. all of the above.   ____

17. As educators we expect our students to succeed, and in the same way we should teach learners to expect:
    a. positive outcomes.
    b. negative outcomes.
    c. the worst; then they won't get disappointed.
    d. never to be as successful as owners.   ____

18. Filling ourselves with positive emotions and attitude leaves no room for:
    a. anxiety.
    c. stress.
    b. fear.
    d. all of the above.   ____

19. Being in a good place emotionally changes the body's production of hormones and antibodies and causes us to:
    a. have accidents.
    b. be anxious.
    c. become ill.
    d. be happier and more energetic.   ____

20. When asking questions about their perspective on life, learners need to reflect upon:
  a. how they face roadblocks.
  b. their negativity or optimism.
  c. whether they are healthy or sickly.
  d. all of the above. ____

21. To improve expectations for success, learners need to expect the best by:
  a. practicing optimism.
  b. surrounding themselves with negativity.
  c. watching sad movies.
  d. eating junk food. ____

22. Confirmations of true statements that are recited daily and help manifest a more positive reality in our lives are referred to as:
  a. admissions.   **c.** affirmations.
  b. denials.   **d.** refutations. ____

23. As educators we can model winning behaviors for our students, such as:
  a. practicing praise.   **c.** counting blessings.
  b. being well.   **d.** all of the above. ____

24. A powerful technique that can move us toward where we want to be in life is:
  a. life skills.   **c.** road mapping.
  b. goal management.   **d.** flow charting. ____

25. In order to fulfill what is required of us in goal management we must have:
  a. self-discipline.
  b. permissiveness.
  c. sanctions in place.
  d. the ability to relinquish our values. ____

26. Winners who effectively manage their goals experience:
  a. less stress and anxiety.
  b. better concentration and job performance.
  c. more happiness than those who do not.
  d. all of the above. ____

27. If students are having problems with goal management, they should ask:
    a. Is it moral, legal, and fair?
    b. Do they want it or is it what their parents want for them?
    c. Is there an emotional commitment?
    d. all of the above. _____

28. In order to achieve our goals we must be patient, plan, and take action. Often it is the:
    a. spreading ourselves too thin, trying to attain too many goals at once, that prevents someone from goal attainment.
    b. inability to stay focused that prevents someone from goal attainment.
    c. fear of failing that prevents someone from goal attainment.
    d. all of the above. _____

29. We instill in learners that the goals they set for themselves must be believable and that learners must:
    a. visualize achieving them.
    b. write them in a book.
    c. carry them around and read them often.
    d. share them with friends. _____

30. When learners are setting goals, the master educator will continue to stress that:
    a. long-range planning is not required.
    b. hard work is all it takes.
    c. success is not passive.
    d. goals must be kept in your head. _____

31. To set up a goal system that will work, your goals must be:
    a. specific and relevant.
    b. measurable and time-based.
    c. attainable.
    d. all of the above. _____

32. Goals are considered long term if they are set to be achieved in:
    a. more than five years.
    b. one to five years.
    c. less than one year.
    d. none of the above. _____

33. When students are reviewing the strategies of effective goal management, they should consider:
   a. their definition of success or failure.
   b. whether their parents are helping them.
   c. whether their friends will commit to help them.
   d. waiting around for the right moment. ____

34. Students committed to act on their goals should consider:
   a. setting deadlines; if you don't meet them it's not important.
   b. taking ample time; if you rush you may not be prepared.
   c. writing down short, intermediate, and long-term goals and dividing them into workable segments.
   d. putting the blame on others if you have enlisted their support; they probably sabotaged the project from the start. ____

35. A mnemonic acronym for success in goal management is:
   a. LATCH.   **c.** BROM.
   b. SMART.   **d.** CABAL. ____

36. It is prudent to periodically review and update your goals; as you grow your ideals will change. It is also proven that:
   a. expecting perfection only leads to disappointment and failure.
   b. failing to achieve a goal is an indicator to abandon these goals and set other, easier to attain, goals.
   c. if you set your goals too high you will fail.
   d. if you have a deficit in your skills you can't fix it once you've begun working on your goal. ____

37. When schools across the country were surveyed, _____ was listed as the most important educator characteristic.
   a. strong work ethic   **c.** accountability
   b. precision   **d.** leadership ____

38. Master educators must provide the industry with trained workers who possess strong occupational skills and good work ethics as well as:
   a. interpersonal skills.   **c.** internal motivation.
   b. positive attitudes.   **d.** all of the above. ____

39. To be considered a winner in an organization, the employee:
   a. shows up, on time, ready to work.
   b. will gripe about the employer.
   c. will come in late and leave early.
   d. will not associate with other employees. ____

40. For our students to develop a strong work ethic, students and graduates will:
- **a.** make a plan; create a "to-do" list of everything to accomplish.
- **b.** set the alarm clock; be consistent with the plan.
- **c.** build stamina; get exercise.
- **d.** all of the above. ____

41. A person whose behavior is imitated by others and who has a strong work ethic that the learner would like to emulate would be referred to as a:
- **a.** hero.
- **b.** role model.
- **c.** paragon of virtue.
- **d.** champion. ____

42. When faced with a problem, do your best to be a problem solver and:
- **a.** don't look colleagues in the eye.
- **b.** only speak to certain peers.
- **c.** practice active listening.
- **d.** use information against others. ____

43. The best way to meet deadlines is to:
- **a.** pretend that they don't exist.
- **b.** never make any.
- **c.** ignore them.
- **d.** be persistent and stick to your projects. ____

44. Getting up in the morning to go to a job you do not enjoy is unpleasant; it is easier to love what you do. To get the job you love and keep it:
- **a.** be a risk taker.
- **b.** be ambitious.
- **c.** take pride in your work.
- **d.** all of the above. ____

45. The beauty industry is one of the most powerful professions in the world, and the people we serve are our:
- **a.** responsibility.
- **b.** asset.
- **c.** profit and losses.
- **d.** charges. ____

46. Our customers, including our students, should be given special treatment so that they will look forward to coming back. To retain clients we must make them feel that:
- **a.** they are dependent on us.
- **b.** they are the purpose of our work.
- **c.** they are interrupting our day.
- **d.** the client is never right. ____

47. Customer service is more than good hair, skin, and nail care; it includes:
    a. client focus; they are the purpose of our work.
    b. the courteous and attentive treatment that we give our clients.
    c. treating our clients like ourselves, with the same feelings and emotions.
    d. all of the above. ____

48. All clients who come into the school should feel special; if treated in such an extraordinary manner the clients:
    a. will feel like they have entered the wrong student salon.
    b. will feel perhaps their medication is off today.
    c. will feel special, and we will create loyal clients who will keep returning and tell others.
    d. will feel uncomfortable and choose to leave and not return. ____

49. After working with a client, reflect on the service and evaluate your performance by asking:
    a. Do I make eye contact?
    b. Do I discuss the client's needs?
    c. Am I a good listener?
    d. all of the above. ____

50. A handshake will reveal a lot about you; when shaking hands use:
    a. a dry, firm, full handshake.
    b. a wet handshake.
    c. a soft handshake.
    d. a fingertip handshake. ____

51. Clients will want to return and will feel special when the team
    a. learns client names.
    b. keeps client records accurate.
    c. recognizes first-time clients.
    d. all of the above. ____

MULTIPLE CHOICE

1. The activity and work of a number of people who
   individually contribute toward a common vision is:
   a. a collective.   **c.** teamwork.
   b. a group of educators.   **d.** faculty.   ____

2. Teams approach their work with:
   a. confidence.   **c.** apprehension.
   b. indifference.   **d.** uncertainty.   ____

3. Teams must be comprised of high performers; even if we
   have a small team we must:
   a. be responsive.
   b. focus on quality.
   c. be sensitive to our clients' needs.
   d. all of the above.   ____

4. If one member is performing badly, it is the leader's
   responsibility to:
   a. let the member in crisis go.
   b. motivate and build the self-esteem of the
       member in crisis.
   c. tell the member it will okay and move on.
   d. berate the member in crisis in front of the others.   ____

5. Research shows that team members are searching for:
   a. participation and contribution.
   b. results and challenge.
   c. responsibility and standing still.
   d. all of the above.   ____

6. Good team leaders will recognize that the team will have
   needs, and that their job as leaders is to:
   a. have their own agendas.
   b. respond positively to the members.
   c. forget the motto "all for one and one for all."
   d. have the members answer to each other.   ____

7. Team leaders will help all members see the best in themselves, which will:
   a. cause disharmony.
   b. cause anxiety.
   c. provide stimulus for great performance.
   d. cause confusion. ____

8. Team leaders will take great care of the team and will go great lengths to understand the qualities of the team; therefore, leaders must have qualities such as:
   a. being trustworthy.
   b. modeling superior customer service.
   c. being a change agent.
   d. all of the above. ____

9. A true leader wants feedback from the team and therefore:
   a. creates meetings annually.
   b. seeks input regularly from team members and follows through.
   c. is out of the office and does not take calls.
   d. just gives lip service. ____

10. A dynamic team leader will encourage members of the team to take risks; this can be a frightening prospect but a true leader will:
    a. turn any mishap into a lesson learned and laugh at a mistake.
    b. use any mishap to berate the member.
    c. betray the trust earned of members.
    d. discourage the members from taking risks. ____

11. Members of the team should see their team leaders:
    a. making fun of the client.
    b. talking about another colleague.
    c. giving outstanding customer service.
    d. speaking ill of their employer. ____

12. For a team to operate at optimal performance, all members must do their job; team leaders will ensure this by:
    a. keeping relevant issues to themselves.
    b. keeping the team in the know on all relevant issues.
    c. letting all rumors continue.
    d. reprimanding those who gossip and backbite. ____

13. Everyone likes to be acknowledged; the team leader with an understanding of the dynamics of team building will:
    a. acknowledge publicly those deficient in customer service.
    b. describe a situation that is obvious to those present, to embarrass a team member and prevent the team from continuing a dialogue.
    c. recognize all members by name and disclose their performance records.
    d. reward performances and use powerful examples of where the team excels and where there are weaknesses, thus promoting open dialogue. ____

14. A brief statement of the purpose of the school or institutions is referred to as a(n):
    a. mission statement.   c. advertisement.
    b. slogan.   d. campaign. ____

15. It has been said that for members of a team or company to put aside their personal agendas they must:
    a. believe in the purpose of the team.
    b. be motivated to achieve the desired results.
    c. hold ownership in the team.
    d. all of the above. ____

16. A mission statement should communicate the essence of your organization to your members and the public in:
    a. one or two sentences.
    b. two or three sentences.
    c. three or four sentences.
    d. four or five sentences. ____

17. If a work team has developed a team mission statement that mirrors the mission of the institution and reflects its own individuality:
    a. it is just another class.
    b. it is fostering competition.
    c. it is building team spirit.
    d. all of the above. ____

18. The team's mission statement should be clear and:
    a. say who you are and what you do.
    b. concise.
    c. state who your customers are.
    d. all of the above. ____

19. When the team reaches its goal in a particular time frame it is cause for:
   a. celebration and reward.
   b. nothing special.
   c. a promotion.
   d. students to be passed over. ____

20. When the team works cohesively the result is:
   a. negative.
   b. positive.
   c. indifference.
   d. none of the above. ____

21. Team members who like each other will participate in:
   a. lack of communication.
   b. condemnation.
   c. mutual support of each other's effort.
   d. altercations. ____

22. In order to build fellowship and camaraderie, successful teams will:
   a. get to know each other better.
   b. socialize together.
   c. design off-site activities.
   d. all of the above. ____

23. Misunderstandings arise in the workplace from time to time; a good leader will use techniques that will resolve conflict by:
   a. ignoring the conflict.
   b. using positive affirmations and active empathy.
   c. letting the members "duke it out."
   d. letting one of the parties go. ____

24. For team members to feel empowered they must be included in:
   a. hiring.
   b. finances.
   c. firing.
   d. decision making. ____

25. Three factors that leaders will consider to ensure a balanced contribution from all team members are:
   a. confidence, exclusion, and empowerment.
   b. confidence, inclusion, and empowerment.
   c. confidence, responsibility, and empowerment.
   d. confidence, passivity, and responsibility. ____

26. Effective responding, rapport building, appropriate business language, negotiating, and consensus building are all part of:
   a. effective communication skills.
   b. multimedia presentations.
   c. audiovisual presentations.
   d. intrapersonal skills. ____

27. An effective leader will take care of the members of the team by presenting them with:
   a. periodic stimulation in the form of a challenge.
   b. too difficult a challenge.
   c. easy challenges.
   d. surprises. ____

28. Taking ownership of the team means that you will take on the challenges and also the responsibility and:
   a. vision.   **c.** authority.
   b. passion.   **d.** humor. ____

29. As in any project that has its members working toward a goal, the final act of recognition sends a powerful message that:
   a. the organization cares.
   b. the team leader cares about good performance.
   c. the team is important.
   d. all of the above. ____

30. An individual's need for growth on a team can be manifest in different ways; one member may desire pedagogical seminars and another may desire field experience. Thus, an insightful team leader:
   a. knows the importance of investing in each team member.
   b. offers only one discounted option.
   c. buys the video presentation for all to see.
   d. chooses for all. ____

31. Effective teamwork is based on:
   a. collaboration and trust between team members.
   b. clear goals and priorities.
   c. good interpersonal relationships and team success.
   d. all of the above. ____

32. Team building can be highly effective in establishing trust and unity among its members; it can be used for:
    a. clarifying shared values.
    b. formulating business strategies.
    c. establishing a vision for the future.
    d. all of the above. ____

33. Communication failure, lack of trust, defensive behavior, irritability, increased conflict, and other negative behaviors are indicative that the team leader should:
    a. perform evaluations.
    b. make team building a priority.
    c. take some members aside for reprimand.
    d. take a much-needed vacation. ____

34. When there is a team-building event taking place, the leadership is interested in gaining the support of the members through their:
    a. purchasing power.   c. "buy-in."
    b. commissions.   d. sales. ____

35. A sound way to obtain student involvement and agreement with rules and projects is referred to as:
    a. the transfer technique.
    b. the control technique.
    c. the alteration technique.
    d. the censor technique. ____

36. The interview is the most popular way to gather data for team building; some other methods include:
    a. auditorium-style seminars.
    b. small-group discussions.
    c. large-group discussions.
    d. essay-type questionnaires. ____

37. Using a team temperature questionnaire will:
    a. uncover the type of team-building necessary.
    b. determine who is the problem.
    c. give a clear picture of the "Gloomy Gus."
    d. all of the above. ____

38. When the team-building event has been planned to make the event successful:
    a. vary the activities.
    b. promote the event weeks in advance.
    c. hold the event off campus.
    d. all of the above. ____

39. During the time team building takes place, one of the events should be:

a. discussion.   c. reiki.

b. meditation.   d. tai chi.   ____

40. Recollection, process, and reflection are of no use if the members do not see any implementation of a plan to document results of the team-building event within:

a. 5 days of the event.   c. 12 days of the event.

b. 10 days of the event.   d. 15 days of the event.   ____

41. When having a team-building event off campus, the leader of the activity should:

a. recognize the efforts of the staff, give them thanks, and give them a token gift at the end of the activity before everyone leaves.

b. ask someone to else to say thank you.

c. pay the bill.

d. thank only those who facilitated and worked on the event.   ____

42. When a lot of effort was expended on the team-building event, a follow-up progress evaluation should be scheduled at:

a. 20-day increments.   c. 45-day increments.

b. 30-day increments.   d. 90-day increments.   ____

43. The evaluation team should consist of:

a. the team leader and team members.

b. the team members.

c. the team facilitator and the team members.

d. the team facilitator, team leader, and team members.   ____

44. When improvement is not being made to the extent expected:

a. the team must work through it.

b. discussion about possible changes should take place.

c. the team must quit.

d. those that are not in agreement should join another group.   ____

45. The best thing about working in teams is that:

a. feeling of fellowship and growth.

b. you build on each other's ideas.

c. two heads really are better than one.

d. all of the above.   ____

CHAPTER 20 Evaluating Professional Performance

MULTIPLE CHOICE

1. The master educator understands the need to remain current in technology and skills as well as the methodologies used to teach that information to learners because:
   a. of the challenges facing them due to varied diversity.
   b. they wish to keep producing successful, knowledgeable, skilled, and competent graduates.
   c. it may be required by state regulations and regulatory agencies.
   d. all of the above. _____

2. Improvement in teaching skills will have a greater impact if:
   a. the educator recognizes the need for a professional development plan.
   b. the evaluation is poor.
   c. the educator sees a video of the lesson.
   d. another educator makes a suggestion. _____

3. When the educator is in the assessment process, feedback will be desired from:
   a. the supervisor and management.
   b. the management and the owner.
   c. students, coworkers, and management.
   d. everyone they come in contact with. _____

4. The purpose of evaluation is to:
   a. cause anxiety.
   b. improve job performance.
   c. keep people on their toes.
   d. find fault with the educator. _____

5. To begin the assessment process the educator must:
   a. identify the areas to be evaluated.
   b. set the criteria for expectations.
   c. adopt a positive attitude toward self-improvement.
   d. all of the above. _____

6. An example of a general standard of evaluation to be reviewed would be:
   a. thoroughness and accuracy.
   b. marital status.
   c. intrapersonal skills.
   d. gender. ____

7. Job performance in regard to production would include:
   a. eliminating nonessential activities.
   b. verifying questionable answers on procedures.
   c. providing a day of work for a day of pay.
   d. meeting commitments as assigned and outlined in the job description and duties. ____

8. Performance based on thoroughness and accuracy would refer to:
   a. paying close attention to instructions and essential details.
   b. working independently with little or no supervision.
   c. maintaining steady performance under work pressure.
   d. developing and displaying self-confidence at all times. ____

9. Performance review in problem solving would include:
   a. evaluating all possible outcomes before taking action.
   b. organizing priorities and following through.
   c. completing assigned tasks and job duties accurately.
   d. maintaining a positive, caring attitude at all times. ____

10. Depending on the organization, the area of job performance dealing with interpersonal skills and professional conduct would review whether the employee:
    a. conducts personal affairs in such a manner that will not reflect negatively on the school or detract from the normal work day.
    b. extends courtesy and respect to coworkers, students, clients, and superiors at all times.
    c. keeps a professional distance and never fraternizes with students; maintains the relationship of advisor, educator, facilitator, and resource person.
    d. all of the above. ____

11. Because all organizations want employees who are
    self-motivated, the performance review in this area will
    determine whether the educator:
    a. maintains memberships in professional organizations.
    b. practices personal business ethics at all times.
    c. respects the property of the institution and takes steps
       to prevent damage to materials or equipment.
    d. initiates prompt corrective actions when goals are not met. ____

12. General standards for work habits might include whether
    the employee:
    a. arrives on time daily.
    b. doesn't leave scheduled classes or duties to take or
       make personal calls; returns calls on scheduled breaks.
    c. provides a day of work for a day of pay.
    d. all of the above.   ____

13. An employee who is cost conscious:
    a. initiates action to solve problems whenever possible
       without supervisory intervention.
    b. sets and meets realistic target dates for project
       assignments.
    c. handles monies responsibly and recovers/restores
       monies lost due to carelessness or mismanagement.
    d. all of the above.   ____

14. "Exercises initiative in starting and following through on
    assigned work" would qualify as a general standard for:
    a. production.
    b. independent action.
    c. work habits.
    d. self-motivation.   ____

15. When the educator organizes and plans work in advance,
    organizes priorities, and follows through, the area of
    performance is:
    a. production.
    b. interpersonal skills and professional conduct.
    c. work method.
    d. problem solving.   ____

16. A list of general tasks or functions and responsibilities to be performed by the educator as needed by the organization is known as:
    a. job qualifications.
    b. necessary guidelines.
    c. summary of duties.
    d. job description. ____

17. Most organizations will present a detailed list of job duties and:
    a. will reserve the right to require additional tasks as deemed necessary by management.
    b. various abilities expected.
    c. levels of knowledge expected.
    d. all of the above. ____

18. A teaching responsibility would be:
    a. follow the school's published curriculum and handouts provided unless deviations are approved.
    b. monitor reception desk activities.
    c. give tours to prospective students.
    d. monitor the parking on the premises. ____

19. Formal performance evaluations are typically covered by:
    a. other colleagues.
    b. supervisory personnel.
    c. students in the upper classes.
    d. the advisory council. ____

20. The responsibility for training educators in the proper procedures and expected behaviors belongs to:
    a. the advisory council.
    b. the state regulatory agency.
    c. Cosmetology Educators of America.
    d. supervisors. ____

21. With regard to performance, other educators are your best resources; they can:
    a. provide useful information in teaching strategies and performance.
    b. report to supervisors of your poor classroom management skills.
    c. rewrite your lesson plans for you to better facilitate efficiency.
    d. assist you in front of the class on the procedures and techniques that need improvement. ____

22. An effective source of educator assessment is the learner who:
   a. will give feedback regarding successful strategies.
   b. is able to comment on relationships established with learners.
   c. sees the handouts and visual aids produced by the educator.
   d. all of the above. ____

23. Learners are a valuable resource when gathering assessment information because:
   a. they cannot be swayed because of prejudices.
   b. they will maintain an objective mind.
   c. learner outcomes may directly relate to the performance of the educator.
   d. all of the above. ____

24. Providing additional resources for the educator to use for support services and educational programs is the:
   a. manufacturer's representative who gives the educator the latest materials.
   b. employer of graduates.
   c. educator content with the status quo who chooses not to move on.
   d. none of the above. ____

25. Recent graduates can give the educator a new perspective on
   a. entry-level skills that are competitive and may relate to the educator's performance.
   b. the number of students who have completed proficiency levels in national testing.
   c. the students who have successfully qualified for state licensing.
   d. all of the above. ____

26. You will continually improve your skills and abilities as a master educator through:
   a. talking to colleagues.
   b. taking classes and seminars.
   c. regular self-assessment.
   d. reading self-help books. ____

27. The feedback from the various evaluation tools will be used to create a:
    a. professional development plan.
    b. professional profile.
    c. professional resource center.
    d. needs assessment. ____

28. Once the objectives and goals have been identified, the educator then can outline the:
    a. time frame.
    b. short-term goals.
    c. strategies.
    d. long-term goals. ____

29. To determine if the plan is working and if the goals and objectives are being met the master educator will:
    a. rewrite the plan.
    b. periodically evaluate the plan.
    c. simply ask the students.
    d. ask other educators. ____

30. The professional development plan should include areas that need improvement; this part of the plan would be stated as:
    a. expected learner outcomes.
    b. strategies and activities.
    c. short-term goals.
    d. a problem area or area of concern. ____

31. The area in the professional development plan that lists specific objectives that are measurable and tie in with the educator's performance is:
    a. short-term objectives.
    b. long-term objectives.
    c. expected learner outcomes.
    d. strategies and activities. ____

32. Behavioral or performance change expected of the learners upon use and implementation of the professional development plan is the area designated as:
    a. short-term objectives.
    b. evaluation of the plan.
    c. long-term objectives.
    d. expected learner outcomes. ____

33. The evaluation of a professional development plan is achieved using:
    a. repeated peer and student evaluations.
    b. notations of personal observations.
    c. student outcomes.
    d. all of the above. ____

34. Master educators will want to continue with their education to:
    a. reacquaint themselves with people they haven't seen in years.
    b. see if other schools are hiring.
    c. stay informed of the changes in technology, products, and tools.
    d. all of the above. ____

35. Continuing education to fulfill professional development may be obtained:
    a. through the National Cosmetology Association.
    b. through the Cosmetology Educators of America.
    c. by attending national trade association workshops and seminars.
    d. all of the above. ____

36. Continuing education events offer educators the opportunity to:
    a. promote serious networking.
    b. share ideas and experiences.
    c. raise concerns over issues relevant to the teaching profession.
    d. all of the above. ____

37. A job description for a master educator will list duties that may change and will include the phrase:
    a. "will perform other tasks as we see fit."
    b. "we, the management, reserve the right to have other duties imposed on the employee."
    c. "and will perform duties deemed necessary by the management."
    d. "will do other jobs that come due." ____

38. Which of the following is an educator's job description?
   a. Never release private information on any student without obtaining written authorization from the student (or guardian/parent if applicable) on the designated form.
   b. Assign clinic students who are not working with clients other course-related activities that do not disrupt other clinic activity.
   c. Properly prepare graduating students for the applicable state licensing.
   d. All of the above. _____

39. An example of a nonteaching duty is:
   a. "must attend staff meetings as scheduled and participate in discussion of all agenda items."
   b. "must keep equipment needed for classroom or clinic instruction clean and in good operating order."
   c. "must write practical or written assignments on the board each day."
   d. "must maintain a thorough, accurate, and current knowledge of the subject matter taught." _____

40. During the formal performance evaluation the supervisor will identify:
   a. strengths exhibited by the educator.
   b. weaknesses needing improvement.
   c. a plan of action.
   d. all of the above. _____

Answer Key

CHAPTER 1

1. d	11. c	21. c
2. a	12. d	22. c
3. c	13. d	23. a
4. d	14. a	24. d
5. b	15. d	25. d
6. a	16. a	26. a
7. d	17. b	27. b
8. d	18. d	28. d
9. d	19. d	29. d
10. b	20. d	30. a

CHAPTER 2

1. a	11. c	21. d	31. b
2. c	12. b	22. c	32. b
3. c	13. c	23. a	33. a
4. b	14. b	24. b	34. c
5. d	15. c	25. c	35. c
6. a	16. b	26. b	
7. b	17. c	27. a	
8. d	18. d	28. d	
9. d	19. d	29. d	
10. a	20. d	30. d	

CHAPTER 3

1. d	11. c	21. d	31. b	41. a
2. a	12. a	22. a	32. c	42. c
3. a	13. b	23. d	33. a	43. b
4. d	14. d	24. b	34. d	44. d
5. c	15. a	25. c	35. d	45. d
6. d	16. b	26. a	36. c	46. a
7. a	17. d	27. b	37. b	47. d
8. a	18. a	28. d	38. d	48. a
9. b	19. b	29. c	39. d	49. a
10. d	20. c	30. d	40. a	50. d

CHAPTER 4

1. b	11. d	21. d	31. d
2. a	12. b	22. d	32. a
3. d	13. d	23. c	33. d
4. b	14. c	24. a	34. b
5. d	15. c	25. d	35. d
6. a	16. d	26. b	36. c
7. d	17. d	27. d	37. d
8. a	18. b	28. c	38. b
9. d	19. d	29. b	39. d
10. a	20. a	30. d	40. a

CHAPTER 5

1. b	11. c	21. b	31. d	41. c
2. a	12. c	22. c	32. d	42. a
3. a	13. d	23. d	33. b	43. b
4. b	14. d	24. d	34. d	44. a
5. d	15. d	25. a	35. b	45. a
6. b	16. d	26. c	36. d	46. a
7. a	17. d	27. d	37. c	47. b
8. c	18. c	28. d	38. a	48. c
9. c	19. b	29. c	39. d	49. c
10. a	20. d	30. c	40. b	50. d

CHAPTER 6

1. d	11. c	21. d	31. c	41. d
2. d	12. c	22. c	32. d	42. d
3. c	13. a	23. b	33. b	43. a
4. a	14. b	24. a	34. d	44. d
5. b	15. a	25. b	35. a	45. b
6. c	16. c	26. a	36. c	46. c
7. d	17. a	27. d	37. b	47. d
8. a	18. b	28. c	38. d	48. c
9. b	19. c	29. b	39. b	49. a
10. d	20. d	30. a	40. d	50. d

CHAPTER 7

1. d	16. d	31. a	46. b	61. a
2. d	17. b	32. b	47. d	62. d
3. a	18. a	33. c	48. b	63. a
4. d	19. d	34. d	49. c	64. d
5. c	20. c	35. d	50. d	65. d
6. d	21. a	36. b	51. a	
7. a	22. d	37. d	52. d	
8. a	23. c	38. a	53. c	
9. d	24. c	39. a	54. a	
10. d	25. a	40. d	55. d	
11. a	26. a	41. c	56. c	
12. b	27. b	42. b	57. d	
13. c	28. b	43. a	58. a	
14. d	29. d	44. a	59. b	
15. c	30. b	45. d	60. d	

CHAPTER 8

1. c	11. b	21. d
2. a	12. b	22. d
3. c	13. d	23. c
4. b	14. c	24. a
5. d	15. b	25. d
6. c	16. b	26. a
7. d	17. c	27. b
8. a	18. a	
9. a	19. b	
10. b	20. c	

CHAPTER 9

1. c	11. d	21. a	31. c	41. d
2. d	12. b	22. d	32. d	42. d
3. a	13. d	23. d	33. d	43. a
4. d	14. c	24. a	34. b	44. b
5. d	15. d	25. d	35. d	45. c
6. b	16. a	26. d	36. c	46. a
7. a	17. b	27. c	37. d	47. d
8. a	18. d	28. b	38. a	48. b
9. c	19. d	29. d	39. b	49. a
10. a	20. d	30. d	40. c	50. d

CHAPTER 10

1. d	11. d	21. d	31. a	41. d
2. d	12. d	22. d	32. b	42. d
3. d	13. a	23. c	33. b	43. a
4. d	14. a	24. b	34. d	44. c
5. a	15. d	25. d	35. d	45. b
6. b	16. c	26. b	36. c	46. c
7. c	17. c	27. d	37. d	47. a
8. a	18. d	28. b	38. c	48. c
9. b	19. b	29. c	39. c	49. a
10. a	20. d	30. d	40. a	50. d

CHAPTER 11

1. c	11. c	21. a	31. b	41. d
2. b	12. d	22. a	32. d	42. a
3. a	13. c	23. d	33. a	43. b
4. d	14. a	24. a	34. c	44. d
5. d	15. d	25. d	35. d	45. b
6. a	16. b	26. a	36. d	46. c
7. d	17. c	27. c	37. c	47. d
8. c	18. d	28. c	38. d	48. d
9. b	19. c	29. d	39. d	49. d
10. a	20. d	30. d	40. c	50. c

CHAPTER 12

1. a	11. d	21. d	31. a	41. d
2. c	12. c	22. d	32. d	42. a
3. b	13. b	23. d	33. c	43. d
4. d	14. a	24. d	34. d	44. d
5. d	15. c	25. d	35. c	45. d
6. c	16. b	26. a	36. c	46. a
7. b	17. b	27. a	37. d	47. c
8. d	18. b	28. b	38. a	48. b
9. a	19. a	29. a	39. d	49. d
10. d	20. c	30. d	40. b	50. a

CHAPTER 13

1. d	16. b	31. a	46. a
2. d	17. b	32. c	47. c
3. d	18. c	33. b	48. d
4. c	19. d	34. d	49. a
5. a	20. b	35. d	50. a
6. b	21. a	36. b	51. d
7. a	22. c	37. d	52. c
8. c	23. d	38. c	
9. d	24. d	39. a	
10. a	25. d	40. d	
11. b	26. c	41. a	
12. d	27. d	42. d	
13. c	28. b	43. b	
14. d	29. a	44. d	
15. a	30. a	45. c	

CHAPTER 14

1. a	11. d	21. d	31. a	41. c
2. d	12. b	22. a	32. b	42. d
3. c	13. c	23. b	33. d	43. a
4. d	14. d	24. d	34. d	
5. a	15. d	25. c	35. d	
6. b	16. d	26. d	36. d	
7. d	17. c	27. a	37. a	
8. c	18. d	28. d	38. d	
9. d	19. b	29. d	39. b	
10. b	20. c	30. a	40. d	

CHAPTER 15

1. a	11. d	21. a	31. b	41. c
2. c	12. a	22. b	32. a	42. c
3. b	13. a	23. d	33. c	43. d
4. a	14. d	24. b	34. d	44. d
5. a	15. c	25. a	35. a	45. b
6. d	16. d	26. d	36. c	46. b
7. b	17. b	27. c	37. c	47. a
8. d	18. a	28. d	38. d	48. c
9. d	19. c	29. d	39. c	49. c
10. a	20. d	30. d	40. b	50. b

CHAPTER 16

1. b	12. b	22. c	32. d	42. b
2. d	13. d	23. a	33. a	43. c
3. a	14. a	24. d	34. c	44. c
4. c	15. b	25. d	35. b	45. a
5. c	16. d	26. d	36. d	46. b
6. d	17. d	27. a	37. d	47. d
7. d	18. a	28. b	38. d	48. d
8. c	19. d	29. d	39. c	49. d
9. a	20. c	30. d	40. d	50. b
10. d	21. d	31. a	41. b	51. a
11. d				

CHAPTER 17

1. d	11. b	21. c	31. d	41. b
2. a	12. c	22. a	32. d	42. b
3. d	13. d	23. d	33. d	43. a
4. b	14. d	24. a	34. d	44. d
5. d	15. b	25. b	35. d	45. c
6. a	16. c	26. b	36. c	46. d
7. c	17. a	27. b	37. c	
8. d	18. d	28. a	38. d	
9. a	19. a	29. d	39. d	
10. c	20. b	30. b	40. a	

CHAPTER 18

1. d	12. d	22. c	32. a	42. c
2. a	13. c	23. d	33. a	43. d
3. b	14. b	24. b	34. c	44. d
4. c	15. a	25. a	35. b	45. a
5. a	16. d	26. d	36. a	46. b
6. b	17. a	27. d	37. a	47. d
7. d	18. d	28. d	38. d	48. c
8. c	19. d	29. a	39. a	49. d
9. d	20. d	30. c	40. d	50. a
10. c	21. a	31. d	41. b	51. d
11. d				

CHAPTER 19

1. c	11. c	21. c	31. d	41. a
2. a	12. b	22. d	32. d	42. b
3. d	13. d	23. b	33. b	43. d
4. b	14. a	24. d	34. c	44. b
5. a	15. d	25. b	35. a	45. d
6. b	16. a	26. a	36. b	
7. c	17. c	27. a	37. a	
8. d	18. d	28. c	38. d	
9. b	19. a	29. d	39. a	
10. a	20. b	30. a	40. b	

CHAPTER 20

1. d	11. a	21. a	31. a
2. a	12. d	22. d	32. d
3. c	13. c	23. c	33. d
4. b	14. b	24. b	34. c
5. d	15. c	25. d	35. d
6. a	16. d	26. c	36. d
7. d	17. d	27. a	37. c
8. a	18. a	28. c	38. d
9. a	19. b	29. b	39. a
10. d	20. d	30. d	40. d